Better Early Than *Never*

A Story of Strength, Courage, and Faith to Face the Impossible

Jenna Tinsley

To my amazing husband who has been by my side through thick and thin. And to my two, sweet miracle babies. You are the joy of my life.

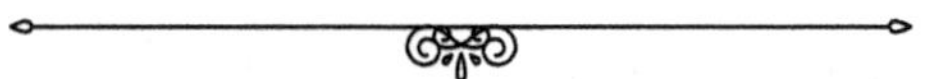

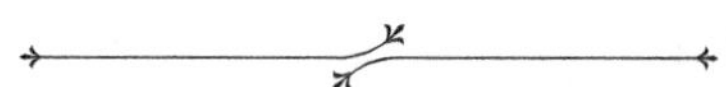

Table of Contents

THE JOURNEY

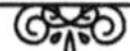

Chapter One

For Better or For Worse

June 2, 2012 was a hot, sunny day in North Texas. I was twenty-seven years old getting ready for another blind date. Completely discouraged by the dating game, I wasn't expecting very much out of this date.

The date was with a guy named Mark. My roommate had given him my number. She met him through a group of friends and thought we might make a good match.

"He's here!" my roommate exclaimed from the living room. His white GMC truck pulled up to the house promptly at ten o'clock. I re-read the text he had sent me the night before, "Pick a color: red, blue, yellow, or green." He had created a date for all the colors and let me choose. I had picked blue, so our date was going to be to the Dallas Aquarium. He came to the door with flowers and a sweet smile. *Maybe this guy would be different from the rest,*

I thought as I checked myself in the mirror before opening the door.

Conversation began in the truck, "Tell me about your family," I asked. He told me about his mom, dad, and two sisters who lived in California. He spoke of them with such fondness. We shared so many things on the ride to the aquarium. Talking with one another was easy. It was as if we had known one another for years. We felt an instant connection.

As we walked through the Dallas Aquarium and enjoyed lunch together afterward, our conversation never stopped. We had so many things in common. We were both involved in the single's ministry, children's ministry, and outreach ministry at the same church. We had both recently been on mission trips to Guatemala. Our groups had gone just a week apart. We had stayed in the same orphanage and knew all the same kids.

Mark had lived down the street from me for years. The house he lived in was on my running path. It was amazing to realize that our paths had crossed so many times and we had never met.

We realized very quickly into our first date that there would be many more dates to follow.

Over the summer Mark and I spent time getting to know one another deeply. The beginning of our relationship was different than many other couples' relationships. It was more pragmatic in nature. Although we loved spending time together, we made a point to see if we would be a good fit for marriage before getting too wrapped up in emotions. We discussed several topics over that time. We explored the topics of faith, roles in marriage, raising children, politics, and lifestyle choices.

By August, it was clear to both of us that marriage was in our future and we fell deeply in love. We had so much fun together. Mark loved to plan fun, exciting dates. I couldn't wait for the weekends to come to see what he had in store for us. We both loved adventure, and we felt care-free when we were with one another. We truly became best friends.

Mark had a calm, sensitive soul, and a deep, soothing voice. I would describe him as more of a "type B" personality. He had an amazing way of calming me down when life seemed to be too much. He was a man of faith, which was something that instantly connected us.

He was a very selfless and caring man. One day when we were heading out to a special date he had planned for us, we came across a stranded driver. His tire had popped, and he didn't have a spare. Mark didn't think twice, he pulled over to help the guy. It took about forty-five minutes to tow the other truck to a car dealership, and make sure he got what he needed. When he got back in the car he was beaming. He always loved an opportunity to help someone. He loved being a hero.

Mark and I had many things in common, but we were also quite different, especially our upbringings.

Mark grew up on twenty-three acres in a small town in Michigan. His high school had a total of eight hundred students. The school included kids from five neighboring towns. His dad was a CNC programmer and his mom was VP Sales for their family sign company. He spent his weekends with his family riding on dirt bike trails and competing in races. He and his two sisters raced dirt bikes until high school. Dirt bike racing was always viewed as a fun experience by his parents. There was never pressure to win or be the best.

I grew up in Albuquerque, New Mexico. I attended a high school with over two thousand students. It was one of thirteen high schools in the city. My dad was a sales broker. My mom was a school psychologist who worked in the public school system. My brother and I had a great childhood filled with a lot of fun, but the main focus of our family was achievement. Whether in academics or sports, hard work and excellence were expected.

Despite our different upbringings, the one thing that connected us more than anything was our strong faith.

We were not ignorant of the challenges of marriage; my parents had recently gone through a difficult divorce. Even so, we were confident that our faith was stronger than anything life would throw at us.

Together, we could handle anything.

* * *

On December 8, 2012, Mark had a special day planned. We had recently returned from a visit to Michigan to meet all his family the week prior. And the night before, he had met my dad for the first time.

He picked me up at three o'clock in the afternoon. His usual calm, relaxed voice was rapid and shaky during the hour-long car ride. We arrived at a campground by the lake. We walked around a bit, enjoying the beautiful fall leaves and the cool, crisp air. Once the sun went down, he led me to a camping spot. Christmas lights illuminated the trees surrounding a picnic table. We sat down at the table and he had made a five-course meal with all my favorite foods. After we ate dinner, he sat next to me, pulled out a ring, and said, "Jenna, you are a treasure and my best friend. The last six months have been the best months of my life. You are truly a gift, and I can't imagine spending my life with anyone else. Will you marry me?"

I eagerly said, "Yes!"

We spent the next hour dancing under the moonlight. We were so in love, and we were confident that nothing would ever change the way we felt about one another.

* * *

The next four months were a whirlwind. We bought a house together. Mark moved into the house first to fix it up, and I planned to move in after the wedding. He was working full time and taking four online classes for his degree. I was busy working, planning a wedding, and decorating our new home.

The big day came on April 27, 2013. Our family flew in from all over the country. The church was beautifully decorated. White bouquets lined the main aisle pews. A large, colorful bouquet sat in the middle of the stage next to a set of three unity candles. The lights were dimmed with *Canon in D* lightly playing in the background. It was all I had imagined it to be.

The music started; everyone was in their seats. Mark walked out with his groomsmen and got in position. Then the doors opened. As I walked towards Mark, a few tears fell from both of our eyes.

The pastor began. "Dearly beloved, we are gathered here today to join Mark and Jenna in holy matrimony." As he spoke, we gazed into one another's eyes. It was as if we were the only two people in the room. Then he got to the vows. We decided to write our own vows. Part of our vows to one another went like this:

"I promise to stick by your side whether this goes really good or really bad because my hope is not rooted in circumstances, it's not even rooted in you, it's rooted in Christ alone, and that can never be shaken."

We read those vows to one another the way most couples read them. We assumed we would only experience the good, and little to none of the bad, especially for the first few years. It was hard to imagine any difficulties between us. We were so in love and got along so well.

"You may kiss the bride," the pastor said. Mark swung me around into his strong arm. He leaned down and we shared our first kiss as a married couple. Everyone cheered. The wedding party and our family exited the auditorium dancing down the aisle to the song, *How Sweet it is To Be Loved By You,* by James Taylor. Then everyone headed to the reception.

The reception hall was beautiful. White, silk linens draped the round tables and chairs. Coral and cream-colored flowers filled the centerpieces at each table, and each chair was wrapped in a silky coral bow. The lights were dimmed, which illuminated the blue, back-lit drapes surrounding the entire hall. In the middle of the room, there was a large, wood dance floor. It was perfect.

We ate, toasted, and danced the night away with family and friends. We exited the reception through two lines of sparklers and headed to a cabin in the woods near Austin. Our honeymoon was so peaceful. We spent the time dreaming about our future. We couldn't wait for our life together to begin and see what God had in store for us.

Chapter Two

Everything We Never Dreamed It Would Be

We decided that we were happy to get pregnant right away after marriage if that is what God would have for us. I had many friends at the time who had struggled to get pregnant, so I figured it would take a while.

It turned out I ended up getting pregnant just seven weeks after our wedding. When we saw the blue line on the pregnancy test, we were ecstatic. It happened a little sooner than we thought it would, but we felt so blessed we were going to be parents.

I found an OBGYN whose office was around the corner from where we lived. He was renown in the Dallas area and had been practicing since the seventies. I knew our sweet baby and I would be in good hands.

My first appointment at eight weeks went great. The baby looked healthy and was measuring right where he or she was supposed to be. All my labs were perfect. My due date was March 25, 2014. *What a perfect time to have a baby,* I thought to myself. The OBGYN seemed confident I would have a normal, healthy pregnancy and delivery.

I decided to find a fun way to announce our pregnancy to our family. I went to the store and bought cards about being grandparents. I put the pictures of our first ultrasound in the card and mailed it to my mom and dad. Then we flew out to California for a vacation with Mark's side of the family. We gave his mom and dad the card in the lobby of the hotel. They screamed so loud in excitement I think the entire hotel heard them. Our baby was going to be the first grandchild on both sides of the family. There was so much joy and happiness in the air, I couldn't wait to share our sweet baby with everyone.

Back at home, Mark and I got back to our jobs. I worked in a hospital as a physical therapist. I shared the news with my coworkers, and they all shared in my excitement. Our lunch conversations quickly turned into anecdotes about pregnancy cravings, morning sickness, third trimester difficulties, and birth stories. I felt like I was suddenly part of a new club, a "mom" club, and I loved it.

I was so excited to be a mom. I was a little anxious about labor and delivery, but I calmed my anxiety by researching and planning. A coworker suggested I watch the documentary, *The Business of Being Born.* I was a bit skeptical after watching it, but it did cause me to consider a natural birth. After further research, I concluded I would aim for natural birth without pain medication. I was open to medical intervention if necessary, but I was young and healthy. I had no reason to think anything would go wrong during delivery. I was confident I would be able to have an all-natural experience.

My pregnancy went very smoothly for the first trimester. I had slight nausea and lightheadedness from time to time, but nothing a little snack wouldn't fix. Overall, it was a very easy first trimester and it hardly interfered with my life at all.

We decided to have the nuchal scan at twelve weeks and learned we would find out the gender early. I received a phone call with the results when I was at work one afternoon. Everything looked good and we would be having a little girl. My eyes teared up. I looked down at my growing belly, "You're my little girl in there," I said under my breath. I walked out to the therapy gym, and the patient I was treating at the time was the first to know. She was a sweet, elderly lady and she screeched in excitement. She told me all about her experience with raising her three daughters. It was the happiest time of her life.

When I got home from work that evening, I decorated the whole house in pink. The house was decorated with "It's a girl" balloons and streamers. Classical lullabies were playing in the background. When Mark got home, I jumped into his arms and cried, "We're having a little girl!" We danced in the kitchen to the music into the evening.

We sat down to think of names, and within about ten minutes we had made a decision. Our little girl would be named, Claire Marie Tinsley. I had always loved the name Claire and Marie was a family name on Mark's side. We called our parents and announced the name, they were so excited.

My mom was the first person I called, "We're having a girl, Mom!" I said with excitement. She was overjoyed. She told me that she always loved the name, Claire, for a girl. I said, "Well you must be a mind-reader, because that's what we're going to name her." It made us both laugh.

We were planning to go visit Albuquerque in December to celebrate Christmas. We planned to have a big baby shower in Albuquerque with all our friends and family during that time. She got to planning right away.

I put my hands on my belly. *My sweet baby Claire,* I thought to myself. I began to dream about what she would look like and what kind of personality she would have. I couldn't wait to be a mommy. I dreamed about going on walks in the mornings and going to our local library for "Mommy and Me." I couldn't wait to take her to the park and show her off to all my friends. All I ever dreamed of was coming true, this was going to be the best chapter of my life.

* * *

Life continued as normal until I was eighteen weeks pregnant. I had a difficult day at work that day, and I was eager to get to my appointment that afternoon to get to see Claire on the ultrasound.

When I arrived at the office, I was called back right away. I was greeted by the sonographer with a warm smile. We had gotten to know one another by then and had formed a good friendship. Mark got there just in time to see the ultrasound. She started recording the measurements and got a confused look on her face. She asked both of us to stand up to see how long our legs were. She said the baby's femur was measuring small and wanted to see if maybe it was genetic. I was concerned because I was 5'9" and Mark was 5'10." It wouldn't have made sense for our baby to measure small. I tried to reason that this could be due to short family members on Mark's side. Still, I wasn't convinced everything was okay.

After the ultrasound, we sat nervously waiting for our OBGYN's arrival. When he walked in, he said, "Everything looks great. Your blood pressure and labs are good too. So, that is great news. I am a little concerned about the baby's measurements. Just to be on the safe side, I would like to send you to a maternal-fetal medicine (MFM) specialist."

He didn't seem too worried, so I decided it was probably just a fluke and everything was fine.

Mark and I met at the MFM specialist's office the next week after work. We were called back to a sterile, cold treatment room. The MFM specialist was a tall man with a strong presence. He didn't say much to us when he walked in, he just got straight to work.

He began the ultrasound. He was calling out numbers to his assistant who was frantically writing them down. At the end of the ultrasound, he said, "Things don't look good. Your baby is below the third percentile for growth. This classifies her as having intrauterine growth restriction."

He didn't know specifically why it was happening, but he gave us a long list of possible causes. These causes included chromosomal abnormalities, birth defects, infection, and a blood clotting disorder. He said that the prognosis was poor because it was so early in the pregnancy to see such severe growth restriction. Because of the lack of nutrients and oxygen to the baby, she had up to a twenty times higher risk of stillbirth. If she did survive, she was ten times more likely to have neurological damage. She would also have a greater likelihood of developing adult illnesses, such as diabetes and hypertension. He told us, "Come back in a week." Then he left.

I sat in my car after the appointment and started crying. I was so confused and scared. *He has to be wrong. It was probably just a problem with the ultrasound machine, or a wrong measurement*, I thought to myself. I had seen many misdiagnoses in my time in healthcare. I assured myself that he was making a big deal out of nothing and trusted that our baby would be fine.

Mark and I decided we did not like the specialist's bedside manner. We told our OBGYN that we would rather see him every week instead. Our OBGYN told us that the specialist's partner was nicer to work with, but we insisted. He reluctantly agreed because there was no other MFM specialist in the area that we could see. He told us if I ended up in the hospital before my due date, they would be our only options. I immediately brushed off his comment. I was certain that this would soon be revealed to be a misdiagnosis, and everything would turn out fine. I knew I wouldn't end up in the hospital early. I was certain I would get the natural, full-term delivery I was planning on.

We went in every week after that. Although she continued to be growth restricted, she was still moving around well. "As long as the both of you are doing well, we will keep her inside of you as long as we possibly can," my OBGYN said at my twenty-week appointment. I asked him if there was anything I could do to help the situation, but he said there was nothing I could do to make her grow any faster.

* * *

By the time I was twenty-three weeks pregnant, Mark and I flew to California for Thanksgiving. We took the red-eye flight and I felt uncomfortable on the plane. It was hard to describe how I felt, I just didn't feel right. We spent four days at his parents' house, and I had a sharp pain on the right side of my abdomen throughout the trip. I ignored it, attributing it to the stress of traveling or something I ate.

When we returned home, I felt really strange, the same way I had felt on the plane. I decided to take my blood pressure because I thought it might be too low. I sat down and relaxed as the cuff inflated, then deflated. It read 180/120. Normal blood pressure is below 120/80. I immediately decided my cuff must be broken. I called the after-hours number just to be on the safe side. They asked if I was experiencing any symptoms, such a headache or blurry vision. I said, "No." The nurse told me to rest and call my OBGYN's office first thing in the morning.

I woke up the next morning and checked my blood pressure again. Again, it read 180/120. I decided to check my blood pressure at work before calling my OBGYN's office. I didn't want to make a big deal out of it. I was certain the problem was with the blood pressure cuff.

When I got to work that morning, I grabbed the blood pressure machine from the gym. I went into the office, sat down, and took it again: 160/110. I called my doctor's office and the nurse said to come in right away. When I arrived at the office, my blood pressure continued to rise. My doctor was concerned that it had elevated so quickly. He sent me to the hospital for monitoring.

At the hospital, they were able to get my blood pressure down with medication, and my labs all looked good. They gave me a steroid shot just in case I ended up delivering early, as it would help strengthen the baby's lungs. My doctor said I had gestational hypertension. He wanted me to take it easy at home and keep up with our weekly appointments. He said that it would be very likely I would deliver a premature baby. I, however, was completely convinced we would go full-term. I even went home that day and signed up for a natural birthing class.

I was in complete denial.

* * *

My weekly appointments went as good as could be expected for the next two weeks. At the end of my twenty-six-week appointment, I met with the check-out person to make the next week's appointment. My appointments usually fell on a Thursday every week. My twenty-seven-week appointment would fall on the week of Christmas. Because of this, they had to squeeze me in on Tuesday morning (Christmas Eve).

A few days before Christmas Eve, I was feeling pretty down. I was really looking forward to going back home for Christmas. I had been waiting so long to celebrate this little girl in my belly with all my friends and family, and Christmas was always such a special time with my family. Mark could tell I was getting tired of this situation. "I'm going to plan a special date for us on Christmas Eve," he said, "we need to have some fun." He started planning somewhere we could go where I could still take it easy.

Christmas Eve came and we headed to our ten o'clock appointment. The sonographer began the ultrasound. Our sonographer was a sweet, bubbly woman who I grew to love. She was always chatty during our appointments. She loved to point out everything she saw on the ultrasound. This morning she was silent. Her face was flat. I waited for what seemed like hours for her to say something.

"Have you felt the baby kick today?" she asked.

"Yes . . . I'm sure I did," I replied.

"I'm just going to call the doctor in to take a quick look," she said.

My heart started to race. She never called the doctor in, why would she need to do that? Then I feared the worse. *Had we lost her?*

"Have you felt the baby kick today?" my doctor asked kindly after looking at the ultrasound.

"Yes, definitely," I replied, questioning my sanity. He asked the sonographer to bring up the heartbeat. To my immediate relief, we heard a heartbeat. It was slow and weak sounding, but it was a heartbeat. My doctor said we needed to go to the hospital right away. The baby was not doing well, and we needed the specialist to take a look. "You need to know this is very serious. The baby may not survive. We will do all we can," the doctor said as we were leaving the room.

We arrived at the hospital and were taken to a triage room. *Oh good, triage*, I thought, *that's not serious*. A sweet nurse strapped a monitor to my belly and told me to relax. She said that they would monitor for an hour and then come back and let me know how it looked.

Then she left the room.

Mark and I were hanging out leisurely, talking about our special date that night. I was sure everything would be fine. Mark stepped out to use the restroom.

Suddenly, three nurses came running into the room. One of them grabbed my left arm to start an IV. The other told me to roll onto my side frantically moving the monitor around on my belly. The third one handed me a pen and told me I needed to sign a consent form for a c-section. I started crying and said, "No, it's too early, I'm not signing."

Just then, Mark came back in and very sternly told them they needed to stop and tell us what was going on. The nurses slowed down and showed us the monitor. The baby's heart rate was decreasing when it should have been increasing, and it was a sign she was in distress.

My OBGYN entered the room and I was so relieved. I was sure he would tell these silly nurses that everything was fine, and it was way too early to deliver my baby. He brought the MFM specialist with him (he brought the nice one he had told us about). The specialist performed an ultrasound. "You see how she's not moving very much? And the amniotic fluid is extremely low? That means your baby has reached a point where she can't survive inside of you anymore," he explained. "Don't worry, this hospital has the top Neonatal Intensive Care Unit (NICU) in the area. Your baby will be in good hands."

Just then my blood pressure cuff inflated, then deflated, and the reading popped up on the screen: 200/130. Everyone looked at the number, then looked at me.

I took a breath and said, "Okay, I trust you. I'll sign the consent." After I signed the paper you would've thought someone sounded a fire alarm. Everyone started rushing around as fast as they could. I was taken to the operating room and given an epidural. The anesthesiologist tried to take my blood pressure and it blew up so much it popped off my arm and fell on the floor. His eyes got wide and he said, "We need to hurry guys."

I started shaking uncontrollably. I was so scared; everything was happening so fast. My doctor entered the room, came over to me, and said, "It's okay. You're almost done. You can do this." Then Mark came in with a surgeon cap on. He came right by my side and put his hand on my head.

I could feel everything they were doing during the ten-minute surgery. It wasn't painful but feeling someone move your organs around is a very strange sensation. I could feel the minute she was out and they cut the cord. I felt immediate relief and relaxation flood my body. Our little girl was born at 2:51 pm at twenty-seven weeks gestation.

I listened for a cry, anything, to know she was okay, but all I heard was silence.

As they were sewing me up, the NICU team rolled an incubator over by my head. "Say hello to your baby girl," one of the nurses said. I got a brief look at her, and then they quickly rolled her out of the room.

* * *

After delivery, I was rolled into a post-op room with my husband by my side. They had given me morphine after the delivery to help with the pain as the anesthesia wore off. The NICU doctor came in after a few minutes. He was a kind, soft-spoken man. I was feeling very out of it from the morphine, and I was having a difficult time focusing on his face and what he was saying. Through the blur, I was able to make out most of what he said:

"Hi Mr. and Mrs. Tinsley, I am the doctor in charge of your daughter's care. At the time of birth, she weighed five hundred grams, which is equivalent to 1 lb. 2 oz. This classifies her as a micro-preemie. We have her stabilized now, but she is in for a difficult night. I need you to understand the possibility that she may not survive these first few days. If she does survive, she will be at high risk for things like cerebral palsy, autism, and developmental delay. I want you to know that our team of doctors and nurses are going to do everything in our power to save her life and lower the possibility of these risks. We will keep you updated throughout the night tonight and you should be able to see her tomorrow."

Once he left, my husband looked at me and grabbed my hand. He didn't have to say anything, we knew this wasn't good.

After about an hour they transferred me to a postpartum room to recover. After getting settled, Mark went out to run a few errands. When he came back, he had bought Christmas lights to decorate our hospital room. Then we called our families and delivered the news. Nobody really knew what to say.

After hanging up the phone, reality finally hit me. I broke down sobbing into Mark's arms. This was not how it was supposed to go. We were supposed to be holding our big, chubby newborn safely our arms. We were supposed to be studying her little face and figuring out who she most resembled. Our room should have been full of family and friends admiring our beautiful baby girl.

Instead, our room was empty. Our one-pound little girl was fighting to survive. She had tubes down her throat, monitors beeping, and strange voices all around her. She had been alive for five hours at that point and had never seen her mommy and daddy. *Was she in pain? Was she being comforted? Did she know how much I loved her?*

My sorrow was immediately interrupted by intense abdominal pain. We called the nurse in and she said it was normal to experience strong pain. The anesthesia had worn off and I was experiencing post-labor contractions. She said that the first night would be the worst. She gave me some pain medication and Mark and I went to sleep.

The nurse wasn't kidding about the pain. I hardly slept at all the first night. When I did manage to fall asleep, I was interrupted by either a nurse taking my vitals or the NICU staff giving me updates on Claire. She was having a lot of ups and downs the first night. They were trying to stay positive, but I could hear in their voices that they didn't have a lot of hope.

Our little girl was in for the fight of her life.

We needed a miracle.

Chapter Three

Tiny but Mighty

Claire had made it through her first night and she was stable.

The nurse came in with a wheelchair and said, "Are you ready to meet your daughter?"

I enthusiastically said, "Yes!" I got out of bed as fast as my post-surgery self could. As we were rolling down the hallways, I had a rush of emotions. I was so excited to see her, but also fearful. I had no idea how to prepare myself for what I was about to see.

As they were rolling me through the NICU, I saw groups of pods. Each pod contained two incubators and one overseeing nurse. There were separate rooms there too. "Those are for the babies who are here for a long time," my nurse explained. I had a feeling my baby would end up in one of those rooms.

I was rolled to one of the pods in the back. A sweet, cheerful woman came over to me. "I'm the nurse in charge of your daughter's care," she said. "She had a hard night last night, she kept us all busy, but she's doing better today. She's definitely a fighter."

I was rolled up to the glass. Inside was my tiny baby.

She was about one foot long.

Her arms and legs were so skinny, skinnier than my pinky finger. Her skin was so thin you could almost see through it. She had a tube coming out of her mouth that was attached to the ventilator machine, which was breathing for her. She also had several other tubes and wires coming off her little body.

My first emotion was overwhelming love. She was moving and acting just like a newborn baby would. It was amazing. I looked at her little eyes, her little nose, her little blonde hair. She was so precious. I knew no matter what happened in the future that I would love her forever.

Then a rush of emotion hit. The tears started falling uncontrollably. I watched her little lungs going up and down like every breath was a battle. She looked exhausted. I wondered if she would be able to keep up the fight. I would have done anything at that moment to change positions with her. I couldn't understand why she was suffering so much when I felt fine. The guilt began to hit hard.

"Okay, we need to place a central line," I heard someone say over my shoulder. Three nurses appeared over the incubator. "I think it would be best that you head back to your room and come back later. You're not going to want to watch this," one of them said to me.

My nurse quickly grabbed my wheelchair and started rolling me out. The tears started flowing again and she handed me a tissue. "I know it's hard, "she said, "No one would ever want to watch their baby have to endure this. I promise these are the best NICU doctor and nurses around. Your baby is in good hands. Hang in there."

* * *

The next few days were spent recovering. My blood pressure was still high, and the nurses wanted me to rest as much as possible. I was able to see Claire a few more times, but they were all very brief visits.

After three days in the hospital, I was discharged home. We packed up our room and I was wheeled downstairs in a wheelchair. Mark went to get the car and I said goodbye to my sweet nurses.

I was getting out of the wheelchair and into the truck. I looked over and saw another woman being wheeled outside to meet her husband. She was holding a chubby newborn with several "It's a girl" balloons tied to her wheelchair. Her husband greeted her with a kiss and they both smiled at their new baby.

I felt like I was punched in the gut. *That's how it's supposed to be*, I thought to myself. Mark and I drove home with an empty car seat in the back of the car and left our tiny baby behind us.

* * *

After being sent home, Mark went back to work. My focus became my own recovery and visiting Claire as much as possible. My recovery from the pregnancy wasn't easy. It took about four weeks for the pain from the c-section to go away completely, and it took six weeks for my blood pressure to return to normal. But whenever I saw my little girl struggling in her incubator, my struggles seemed like nothing compared to what she was enduring.

I spent most of my days in the NICU after I was discharged. I was so grateful to live only a few minutes from the hospital and to not have to go to work.

The days were long and difficult at the hospital. A fellow preemie mom told me, regarding the NICU, "They tell you it will be a roller coaster ride, but they fail to mention you're being dragged by your heels."

There were so many emotional ups and downs throughout the day. The mood could change instantly based on how your baby was doing. For the first few weeks, Claire could be doing well one minute and awful the next. My eyes were opened to a whole new world full of sadness, joy, exhaustion, frustration, and peace all within a ten-minute span.

I was so thankful to be introduced to two women who had been in my shoes not long before me. I met them a few weeks after Claire was born. One of them had a twenty-eight-week preemie girl who weighed 1 lb. 12 oz. at birth. The other had a twenty-four-week preemie boy who weighed 1 lb. 2 oz. at birth, just like Claire. The two women were one of the biggest gifts I was given during our preemie journey. Being able to talk to someone who understands what you are going through during a difficult time is a priceless treasure.

I will always be grateful for them.

* * *

Claire survived her first three weeks of life. She was slowly gaining weight and was stable. She still required a ventilator to breathe for her since her lungs were too immature to breathe on their own. She had a feeding tube because she was too young to eat on her own. Due to her first few nights being so difficult, she was at high risk for bleeding on her brain, which can lead to cerebral palsy. She would need at least two CAT scans of her brain before leaving to make sure there were no bleeds.

The first few weeks were spent sitting by her incubator and watching over her. I was hopeful that just my presence in the room would bring her comfort and help her fight.

The NICU required sound and physical touch to be kept to a minimum. This is because a premature baby's nervous system is immature, and they cannot handle noises and touch like a full-term baby can. There were designated "touch times" every three hours. During these times, the nurse and I would open little "doors" on her incubator. These "doors" were small, circular openings just large enough for our hands to fit through. I would help change her diaper and take her temperature. The first time I did this I was terrified. Her legs were so little I thought I would break her, but over time it became more comfortable. After the diaper change and temperature check, I would be able to place my hand firmly over her for a few minutes. Premature babies' nervous systems cannot handle soft touch. Every touch needed to be firm.

The day came when she was about three weeks old that I finally got to hold her. Mark took off from work to experience it with me. He brought a camera to film the event. When everyone was ready, I sat in a recliner next to her incubator. It took four nurses to get all her cords situated. One of the nurses pulled her out of her incubator, turned her carefully onto her tummy, and placed her on my chest. My heart exploded with love and joy the instant she was finally in my arms. She was so tiny, her entire body fit on my chest. Her little hand was moving up and down on my neck. I was in love.

Once they got everything in position and she was stable, they left Mark and me to be with her. I looked around at all the monitors and machines and took in the reality of the moment. My joy quickly turned to tears. I was fearful to move because even the slightest movement could cause one of her tubes to be pulled out. I hated this situation so much. This was not at all how holding your baby for the first time was supposed to be. Mark wiped my eyes and smiled as he looked at her. I decided to focus on joy. Our little girl was alive and thriving. That was something to be celebrated.

* * *

Claire's little personality came out over those first few weeks of her life. She was a feisty little thing, which is probably how she survived all she had to go through. She absolutely hated being put on her tummy. One day I came in and the nurse came to me. "You won't believe it, she rolled over from her tummy to her back last night!" Apparently, she was so mad to be in that position she just rolled herself over. The nurses were shocked to see such a small baby do that. They started calling her, "The NICU gymnast."

When Claire was four weeks old, the doctors began trying to wean her off the ventilator since she had been on it for so long. The ventilator had the potential to cause permanent lung damage, which could affect her for the rest of her life. The longer she was on it, the higher the risk of damage, so they wanted to wean her off it as soon as possible. It was heart-wrenching to watch them try to progress her off the ventilator. I would sit by her incubator and watch her oxygen saturation on the monitor. I would watch it drop over and over and feel defeated as they told me she's not ready and would have to put her back on the ventilator.

They performed an ultrasound after several unsuccessful attempts to wean her off the ventilator. They found that her patent ductus arteriosus (PDA) hadn't closed. The PDA is a hole in the heart that allows the heart to bypass the lungs while a baby is in the womb. It usually closes on its own after birth, but many times a premature baby's PDA does not close. We were told that the unclosed PDA was preventing her from weaning off the ventilator, and we had a difficult decision to make. They gave us two options. First, we could give her one more week to see if the PDA closed on its own. But that would increase the risks that come with more time on the ventilator. The other option would be to perform surgery to close the PDA. She would need to be put under anesthesia and the surgery came with multiple risks. One risk being permanent damage to her vocal cords.

They needed a decision quickly, so I stepped out and called Mark. It was such a difficult decision. Both options came with long-term risks, but we had to choose. These were the types of decisions we ended up needing to make several times during our time in the NICU. Decisions that had no good solution. Either way, we were looking at long-term problems. We had to choose the lesser of two evils.

We talked for a few minutes and told them our decision: we would go forward with heart surgery.

I hardly slept the night before her heart surgery. My mind raced with whether we were making the right decision or not.

When we arrived the next morning at the hospital, they closed the entire NICU down. They did this to create a sterile environment for Claire's surgery. All the nurses and doctors were wearing gowns and surgical masks.

They allowed us to go in and see her briefly as they prepped her for surgery. I looked down at our little baby, who now weighed exactly two pounds. The surgeon came over to talk to us. He was a very charismatic man with a strong presence. "Hi, I'm the surgeon that will be performing your daughter's surgery today," he said. "First we will be putting her under anesthesia. Once she's asleep, we'll make a slight cut under her armpit. Then we are going to take a small clamp and move it inside of her body. We will weave it around her lungs, clamp her PDA, then pull it out."

He had magnifying goggles on his head that he would use to watch and make sure the probe was going where it needed to go. It would only take about ten minutes after the first cut. He explained the risks but assured us that they had done this procedure many times and not to worry.

Mark and I stared at him speechless. *You're going to do what?* I thought to myself. *How was it possible to weave around a two-pound baby's lungs and not hit something?* I wished that he had not explained the procedure, I would have rather not have known.

Mark and I went out to the waiting room as they began the procedure. "God, please protect our little girl," we both prayed together holding hands. Then we sat and waited.

We waited for what seemed like hours. In reality, it was only about forty-five minutes from start to finish. The doctor came out and told us that the surgery was successful, and we could go in and see her.

I was so relived she was okay but couldn't help but think of how it would affect her in the future. Something we wouldn't know for a long time. For the moment, we just had to keep focusing on keeping her alive.

We had to trust that we would be given the strength to handle whatever was given to us in the future.

* * *

The next few days revealed that the surgery was a success. She was able to completely wean off the ventilator and transfer to the much gentler CPAP machine. The CPAP basically assisted her breathing if she needed it, but she did most of the work. I was so relieved to stop the damage the ventilator was doing to her little lungs.

Once the ventilator was removed, we were finally able to hear her sweet little cry. We heard it for the first time as Mark and I were getting ready to give her a bath. He quickly grabbed his camera. My eyes filled with tears. I finally got to hear her sweet little voice. I had been waiting for this day since the day she was born. From that day on, my heart was filled with gratitude every time I heard her cry.

The days after surgery I couldn't hold her. I just spent the time sitting next to her incubator. I would watch her monitors and anticipate the next "touch time." I always looked forward to the moments when she could feel my touch and hear my voice.

One day during that time, I remember looking around and realizing how strange it was to be on the other side of things. I had worked in the ICU for years. I was familiar with all the alarms and monitors. I knew how to distinguish a false alarm from an actual problem, but on this side of things, all I felt was fear and angst. Every time a monitor went off, I shot up in worry. I didn't understand why the nurse wasn't reacting the same way. This experience was certainly giving me a greater understanding of my patients and their families.

One morning, as I was standing over my tiny little baby, my eye caught a glimpse of a stocking next to her incubator. The nurses had made Christmas stockings for all the babies born around Christmas. It was decorated with her name and birthday. I remembered that our weekly appointments were usually on Thursdays, but she was born on a Tuesday because they had to move our appointment that week. The doctor told me that she would not have survived another 24 hours inside of me. *She wouldn't be alive if our appointment wasn't changed,* I thought to myself. That was just the beginning of little miracles we experienced throughout this journey.

* * *

The days rolled on, and Claire was progressing slowly but surely. It was now February. When Claire was six weeks old, she got to move to a private room. I was so excited, I spent an entire day decorating the room. It was nice to be in a room by ourselves. It was a relief to be able to close the door and spend time with my baby alone and to have a small feeling of normalcy.

She was now off the CPAP machine and on to a nasal cannula. The nasal cannula was a tube that was placed in front of her nostrils for her to get extra oxygen. She now was doing all the breathing on her own. I was so happy because I could finally see her sweet, little face. I was able to hold her more often now and helped the nurses give her baths. We even got to dress her in her first outfit. It was fun to be able to feel like I could do more with her and take some responsibility for her care.

The day came when she was thirty-three weeks gestational age that we could begin trying to give her a bottle. They wanted me there for the first feeding and I was so nervous. I had gotten to know several other preemie moms at that point. I learned that premature babies tend to struggle to eat, a problem that can stick with them through their toddler years. This is especially true for preemies who have been on ventilators. The ventilator can affect their gag reflex. It causes the reflex to become more sensitive, which makes it much more difficult to eat.

The first time I tried to feed her she did well for a preemie of her size. Even still, feeding a preemie is not easy. A full-term baby is developed to a point that they can easily figure out how to eat and breathe at the same time. Preemies cannot do this. This causes them to stop breathing completely while trying to eat (which is called apnea). The first time it happened I was terrified. Her little lips started to turn blue and her face turned an ash grey. I called the nurse frantically. She came over, pulled the bottle out, sat her up, and started vigorously rubbing her back. Claire eventually started to breathe again, and I got back to feeding. This would happen two or three times every time I fed her and feeding became an incredibly stressful activity. This was nothing like I had imagined it being. I longed for the day we could bring her home. The day I could feed her gently in her rocking chair in the peace of our home. No monitors, no beeping, no nurses, no fear. I began to wonder if that day would ever come.

* * *

Over the next few weeks, Claire began to do exceedingly well with feeding. The NICU doctor and nurses told me they had never seen a preemie born that small be able to drink from a bottle that well. Mark and I beamed with pride. That was our little fighter.

By late February, she was big enough to get out of her incubator and into an open crib. I could finally pick her up anytime I wanted. I began to really feel like her mom and not just a bystander in her care. It was a wonderful feeling.

In the beginning of March, she had her final CAT scan on her brain. All her CAT scans showed no brain bleeds, which surprised all the doctors and nurses.

One Monday morning in late March, I walked into the NICU and a nurse came right over to me. She was so excited to tell me the news: Claire would be able to come home that Saturday. She would be coming home three days before her due date.

I was so excited but also anxious. I had always had the nurses on the other side of the door in case something happened. Now it would just be us.

I spent that day going over all her discharge information. I learned all about the oxygen tanks and the oxygen monitor she would be coming home with. There was a very specific way to use the oxygen tanks and a protocol for replacing them.

We also had several doctor's appointments scheduled the next week. This included an appointment with a pediatric ophthalmologist. Claire had something called Retinopathy of Prematurity. This occurs when the blood vessels in the eyes do not form correctly, which leads to scarring on the retinas. This can cause visual problems, even blindness, as the baby gets older. It is caused by the supplemental oxygen a premature baby is given in the NICU. The more oxygen the preemie requires, the more severe the retinopathy. Therefore, it is usually more severe in micro-preemies. She would need several eye exams to keep a close watch on it.

The NICU staff allowed us to spend the night at the NICU the night before she was discharged. This would allow us to have complete responsibility for her care, but with the reassurance of the nurses there, in case we needed them.

We arrived at the NICU with our overnight bags. They took us to our room and went over everything we needed to do throughout the night. To say we were overwhelmed is an understatement. There were vitamins, medications, an oxygen tank, and a monitor. She was on a strict feeding schedule every three hours. She required the proper mixture of formula so that she could get extra calories.

"Claire has been sleeping really well at night," said the nurse as she was leaving the room. "I'm sure she won't give you any trouble."

Great! we thought to ourselves. Unfortunately, we were about to have those expectations shattered.

* * *

The night began with getting everything situated and organized. Claire was awake but quiet in her crib. I fed her at nine o'clock at night, and she fell asleep in my arms. I put her in the crib, and we turned out the lights to go to sleep.

About five minutes later we both shot up to the sound of loud screaming and a blaring oxygen monitor. I picked Claire up, rocked her gently and she fell back asleep. I put her into her crib, but the minute I put her down she started crying again. This cycle went on for about two hours. I eventually let Mark sleep for a bit while I rocked her until midnight, which was her next feed.

Mark took the next feed, and by this point, Claire was wide awake. We thought that maybe she was so used to all the lights and noises in her NICU room that she couldn't sleep when it was dark and quiet. We turned on the lights and the TV in hopes that she would go to sleep. It didn't work. She was alert and awake for three hours until her next feed. Then she wouldn't sleep unless she was held.

She continued this cycle until the morning. When the nurse came in at nine o'clock in the morning, she said, "So how'd it go?" Mark and I looked at each other with exhausted eyes. "She didn't sleep as well as we thought she would," I said softly.

"Oh, she probably just has her days and nights mixed up. She'll get it down soon. Don't worry," the nurse said sweetly.

We got everything packed up and said our goodbyes to all the amazing nurses and doctors. We were incredibly grateful for all they did for our baby.

We got in the car, and after eighty-eight long, exhausting days in the NICU, we brought our little girl home.

* * *

When we got home, we took Claire out of her car seat and showed her around. We didn't go upstairs, because to go upstairs we would have had to change her oxygen monitor to the portable tank. It took about fifteen minutes to do that.

We got her and all the things that came with her situated. She slept peacefully in my arms most of the day. We were both so exhausted already and were wondering how we were going to survive without sleep. We had planned for her to sleep in our room at night. We were hopeful that she would sleep better that night than she slept the night before. But we were going to soon learn to set the expectation bar very low for our little girl.

The first night was extremely hard. Claire cried most of the night. When she wasn't crying, her oxygen monitor would slip off her little foot and the alarm would sound. This would cause her to wake up and cry. We decided that if we were going to make it through this, we would need to take shifts. After that first night, we began having one of us out in the living room with her and the other in our bedroom to get some sleep. After three hours we would switch.

The first few days were quite an adjustment. Claire slept well during the day if she was being held. Once the evening came, she began crying. No matter what we did the crying would continue until around one o'clock in the morning. Then, once she finally fell asleep, she would be woken up by the monitor giving a false alarm. Every time that monitor went off, I would shoot up in fear. Neither of us slept much when it was our shift, even if Claire was sleeping. We were so worried something would happen to her.

One morning, a few days after we got home from the NICU, I was feeding Claire in our room while Mark was in the kitchen. Everything was going well with the feeding when suddenly she stopped breathing. Her oxygen monitor started blaring. This had happened in the NICU several times and I knew what to do. I picked her up, put her on my shoulder, and started vigorously rubbing her back. But it wasn't working. I started to panic. My heart was pounding. I immediately jumped out of bed and laid her on the floor. I started rubbing her sternum, a technique I learned in the hospital.

"Please breathe, please breathe," I whispered under my breath. Just as I yelled out for Mark and began to start CPR, she started breathing. I picked her up just as Mark came in.

"She's okay," I said softly.

I sat there with her shaking and crying. *What if she stops breathing in the middle of the night and I'm not there to help her?* This thought led me to obsess over her breathing. I began to wake up several times an hour each night to check that she was still breathing. I couldn't lose her, not after all we had been through.

* * *

The weeks went on and things didn't get any easier. The constant worry and excessive lack of sleep began to put a strain on our young marriage.

The differences between Mark and I began to be exposed more and more. All of that, mixed with the high-stress environment, led to arguments and frustrations. I was having such a difficult time. The achiever in me was hit hard. "Maybe there's really nothing we can do to stop her from crying," Mark would say calmly as we were taking turns bouncing her in the evenings. "Of course there is. There must be a reason she's crying. I'm her mom, I should be able to know what's wrong." I would say frustratingly. This was the first time in my life that I was met with a challenge that I didn't feel confident to handle. I had no idea what I was doing. I felt so overwhelmed.

Mark didn't have the advantage of spending three months in the NICU learning how to take care of Claire as I did. He was eager to take care of our new baby, but I made him feel like he couldn't do anything right. On top of that, there were many added stressors in his life at that time. He was taking several classes to finish up his degree. Also, his job as a software engineer was in jeopardy. The company where he had worked for the last ten years was cutting back. He hadn't kept up with the current technology, and he was worried he wouldn't be able to find another job. We couldn't put Claire in daycare because of her immature immune system, and we didn't have any family in the area, so one of us had to stay home with her. He was feeling the pressure of needing to provide for our family and was spending many late hours studying for classes and learning about new technologies.

One morning we were sitting on the couch together. We were so tired our bones ached. We had never been so exhausted, so overwhelmed, so stressed. Claire had fallen asleep in my arms and the room was quiet. We looked at each other and for the first time in our marriage, we really saw each other. The facades had fallen off. All the hurts, all the failures, all the imperfections had been brought into the light. At that moment Mark grabbed my hand and gave a slight smile. For the first time in our lives, we both felt fully exposed and fully known. Yet we knew we were fully loved despite our failures and imperfections. We thought we understood love, but now we were beginning to realize what love really was. As we sat holding hands in silence, I knew this wouldn't break us. We were a team, and we were in this together.

* * *

After a few months, things were getting a lot better. Claire was sleeping better at night. Our lives were becoming much less stressful.

She was growing and thriving. She was able to wean from the oxygen after four weeks, and she was able to get off the oxygen monitor after eight weeks. It was an epic celebration in our house the day we said goodbye to that monitor.

We were so impressed by our little girl. She was smiling, cooing, and rolling.

She hit eight pounds after two months and could finally fit into her newborn clothes.

She had to endure a total of nine retinal exams in her first few months of life. Her last exam revealed that her Retinopathy of Prematurity had completely resolved.

Her eyes were perfect.

She was meeting all her milestones on time. Her pediatrician was amazed at her progress and her strength. Most micro-preemies are late meeting their milestones, but Claire was right on track. We were so grateful for her and amazed by our little fighter.

She turned into a sweet, happy baby after the colic passed. She still liked to be held all the time (I nicknamed her my, "Velcro Baby"), but as long as she was being held, she was a joy to be around. She was very chatty and loved singing along to her favorite song, "Let's Get Together," from the movie, *The Parent Trap*. She had a big smile and an infectious laugh. We were so in love.

Because we came home during the flu season, we had to completely lock-down our house. Claire had been diagnosed with chronic lung disease. Her body would most likely not be able to fight even a mild cold. Because we didn't want to take any chances, we decided we would lock-down for her first year just to be on the safe side. We would only allow immediate family to visit, and they were asked to take precautions, such as removing their shoes and using hand sanitizer.

It was a long year being locked inside, and some days were a little lonely. But we did all we could to make the best out of it. I created stations around the house where she could play so she would stay entertained. We waited in anticipation for the trash man to come every week and we had daily trips out to the mailbox. It was just me and my little girl all day and that was enough for me.

* * *

Claire's first birthday was a momentous celebration. I was in tears all day thinking of all she had been through during her first year of life. She was the strongest person I knew, and I was privileged to be called her mommy.

We were still on lock-down on her first birthday, so we had a Skype birthday party with all our family. Claire was now 12 lb. 15 oz. She was crawling, pulling up to stand, and getting into everything. Her smile, laugh, and babbling filled our house all day long. She was our miracle baby, and we spent the day celebrating all the Lord had brought her through.

A few months after she turned one, we were able to get out of lock-down and start exploring the world outside of our home. I had the best time with her. We went on walks with neighbors in the mornings, met friends at the park, and went to "Mommy and Me" at the local library. We got to do everything every other "normal" family got to do.

I finally had the life I had always dreamed of. We couldn't have been happier.

Chapter Four

If at First You Don't Succeed

In the spring of 2016, Claire had just celebrated her second birthday. She was such a sweet, sensitive, joyful little girl. She had wavy, blonde hair and bright, blue eyes, just like her daddy. She was a tiny little thing, she only weighed twenty pounds. But it made her that much cuter. Her calm, sweet disposition made her a very easy toddler. One of her favorite things to do was dress like Mommy. There were many mornings that she would go to my closet and pick out a vest for me to wear. Then she would go to her room and pick out a vest for her to wear. Then she would run to me and say, "Ok Mommy, let's be vest friends today!" It was precious.

She had a bounce to her step and hopped everywhere she went. She woke up in a great mood every day and got excited about the littlest things throughout the day. She radiated happiness and it was contagious.

She absolutely loved other kids. Whenever we would go to the park, I would unhook her from her car seat and set her down on the sidewalk. She then would run as fast as her tiny legs would take her yelling, "Hi kids! Hi kids!"

It was such a joy to get to spend every day with her and see her grow and develop.

She hit every milestone as any other full-term baby would. She wasn't showing any long-term effects of her prematurity. She loved to eat and was the least picky toddler I knew. Every time I watched her eat my heart was filled with gratefulness. I was so amazed and thankful that it wasn't a struggle for her like it was for many micro-preemies.

She was the strongest person I had ever met, and I felt so privileged to be her mommy. We were in a season of joy and happiness as a family of three.

* * *

Around that time, Mark and I began discussing whether we would want to have another child. There were so many things to consider. We thought about Claire being an only child. She would probably be fine, but she loved kids so much and was so social, we knew it would be best for her to have a sibling. There was something in me that felt like we were meant to have two children.

We took a few months to consider all the options and it came down to either natural pregnancy or adoption. Both had pros and cons, it was a difficult decision to make.

I met with several doctors, including my OBGYN from Claire's pregnancy. There was never a clear reason for what went wrong in my first pregnancy, so it was difficult to determine the risk of something going wrong again. I was in excellent health, so I was given the green light from all the doctors to get pregnant again. My OBGYN said that I had a small chance of it happening again, but that we would be more prepared this time. He was prepared to do everything he could to help me have a healthy, full-term pregnancy.

Mark and I spent another month or so praying about it and going through the pros and cons. We came to a point that we were confident of what God wanted us to do and decided to try to get pregnant. We would trust that He would give us the strength to get through whatever would come. In my mind, no matter what happened, it couldn't be worse than my first pregnancy.

*　*　*

We found out I was pregnant again on Father's Day of 2017. We were so excited. I had a strong confidence that this pregnancy would be different from the first. I felt healthy and strong and genuinely believed that we would get a story of redemption. I believed that the fear and anxiety I experienced in my first pregnancy would be replaced with peace and joy in this pregnancy. I believed that I would get the things I so looked forward to during my first pregnancy. I would get to show off my big belly. I would deliver at full-term. My family and friends would be in the hospital room admiring our new baby after delivery. We would bring our big, chubby newborn home a few days after giving birth. No monitors, no beeping, no tubes, no having to ask permission before holding my baby. It would be just what I always wanted, and I was confident this was God's plan.

*　*　*

I was four weeks pregnant when we got a positive pregnancy test. It only took a few days for the morning sickness to hit, and it hit hard. It was much more severe than the first pregnancy. I also felt so different than I did during my first pregnancy. I felt like my heart was racing all the time, even when I was resting. I felt very nervous and sweaty and could not handle being outside in the heat for more than a few minutes. I was also weak and tired all the time. I knew that every pregnancy could be different, so I just assumed it was all a response to hormones. I tried my best not to worry about it.

My nausea increased to vomiting at five weeks pregnant, and it was unrelenting. I would wake up, and the minute I stepped out of bed I would throw up. Then I tried to eat something so I could take all my vitamins and supplements and would immediately throw it up. I began throwing up five to six times a day. I had an underlying intense nausea throughout the day that never subsided. It felt like a combination of the flu and food poisoning, day in and day out. I tried to do things with Claire and give her some resemblance of normalcy, but sometimes all I could do was put on the TV and lie down on the couch. I was so thankful Mark now had a work-at-home job because he could play with Claire during his breaks. It was during that time that I realized what a great man I married.

The day came for my first appointment at eight weeks. I was nervous. A lot of emotions were triggered by going back to the same office where everything went wrong with my first pregnancy. I tried to stay positive and confident that the outcome would be better this time around.

The ultrasound went well. The baby looked good and was growing right on track. But when I went into the exam room and the nurse took my blood pressure, she was shocked. My blood pressure was 160/100. I told her I was nervous, but she said that was way too high for this stage of pregnancy. My OBGYN came in next. He said that he was a little concerned that my blood pressure was already rising. He decided to start me on blood pressure medication again. He told me to monitor my blood pressure at home regularly. We scheduled a 12-week appointment and he said to call if anything came up.

A few days later I had started the medication and it was working well. My blood pressure was at a normal level. I was relieved we were able to bring my blood pressure down, but I still felt awful.

That morning I got a call from the nurse at the doctor's office. I knew it was her since I had her number saved from my previous pregnancy. We knew each other very well by now. When I picked up the phone, she didn't have the normal upbeat sound to her voice. She had more of a worried tone. "Hey Jenna," she said, "we got your labs back and it looks like there might be something going on." My stomach dropped. "Your thyroid function is too high. You need to see an endocrinologist as soon as possible. I've sent your information to an endocrinologist we work with and they will be calling you this afternoon to make an appointment."

We said, "Goodbye," and I hung up the phone. I sat down and stared at the ground. "Where are you, God," I prayed under my breath. "This is not how this was supposed to go. I prayed for you to redeem this pregnancy. Instead, it's going worse."

My appointment was scheduled a few days later. I was so hopeful that the endocrinologist would find an error and tell me that everything was okay. But that's not what happened.

He was a nice and calm doctor. He spent so much time with me, and I never felt like he was in a rush. He did an exam and performed an ultrasound on the front of my neck. Then he took me to his office to sit down and explain what was going on.

I sat there wringing my hands as he spoke. "It is clear from your lab values and the ultrasound that you have hyperthyroidism," he said calmly. "This explains the symptoms of a racing, pounding heart, weakness, anxiousness, and fatigue. This usually is not a very big deal and easy to treat. But because you are pregnant, this is a very difficult situation. Hyperthyroidism only occurs in 0.2% of pregnancies. If left untreated it can lead to miscarriage, premature birth, low birth weight, preeclampsia, and stillbirth." All those side effects sounded all too familiar and my heart sank.

He said that there was a treatment available for pregnant women, but there was a chance it could cause birth defects. He gave me a minute to decide what I wanted to do. Another difficult decision in which I had to pick the lesser of two evils. I felt like I was in the NICU all over again.

"Ok, let's go forward with the treatment," I told him. "The risks of not taking the treatment outweigh the risks of taking it." "I agree and I think you're making the right decision," he said calmly. I checked out and left the office with a heavy heart.

I started the medication and had to trust that God would protect our baby, however, I wasn't as confident as I once was. I lied down after taking my first dose of the medication. I had just put Claire down for a nap and I was feeling extremely nauseated and weak. I laid there taking in the moment. I was only nine weeks pregnant and had an awfully long road ahead of me. I knew that there was a good chance this little baby inside of me may not survive. If the baby did survive, he or she could be born early with birth defects. I felt so scared. I wanted out. I didn't want to have this responsibility.

I closed my eyes and prayed the most heartfelt prayer I had prayed in a long time. "God, this time around, please allow me to take the suffering. The hardest part of our last NICU experience was having to watch Claire suffer. I ask that all the suffering be put on me this time around. Please spare this little baby."

He was about to answer that prayer in a big way.

* * *

Things were the same day in and day out. It felt like such a beat down to be so sick every day. There were days I didn't even want to get out of bed in the mornings because I knew what the day was going to hold. I began to develop huge compassion for those suffering from chronic illnesses. I could not imagine feeling so horrible all day, every day without any end in sight.

One day was particularly bad. I was thirteen weeks pregnant. This is the time during pregnancy when morning sickness is supposed to start subsiding. Mine was getting worse.

I was throwing up constantly that day, and it wouldn't stop. I probably threw up thirty times and couldn't keep anything down. That evening I began to throw up blood, so I called my OBGYN. He told me to go straight to the hospital. I called my sweet neighbor who didn't hesitate to come over and watch Claire for us so we didn't have to wake her up. When I got to the emergency room, I was taken straight back. My blood pressure was 160/110. They gave me an IV with blood pressure medication and anti-nausea medication. I felt instant relief. It was the first time I hadn't felt nauseated for two months. "This is what heaven must be like," I joked to my husband. I then asked the nurses if they could move in with us.

The doctors and nurses in the emergency room were so nice and caring. They gave me some food that I was able to keep down. My labs came back and I was diagnosed with hyperemesis gravidarum. This is a pregnancy complication associated with severe nausea, vomiting, extreme weight loss, and dehydration. At this point, I had lost fifteen pounds since my initial prenatal appointment. They gave me a prescription for anti-nausea medication and told me to hang in there. Then we were sent home.

* * *

My next appointment with my OBGYN was at sixteen weeks. Although I was not doing well, all the ultrasounds up to that point were showing the baby to be doing just fine. This ultrasound was no different. The baby was kicking, moving, and growing right on track. They were able to see the gender and asked if we wanted to know. Claire was with us for this appointment and she excitedly said, "Yes!"

We found out we were having a little boy. It was a moment mixed with joy and worry. We knew from our previous NICU experience that premature boys tend to not do as well as girls. The nurses even have a nickname for white, premature males: wimpy white boy.

When we got home from that appointment that afternoon, I began to pray a Bible verse over our little boy every day:

"Be strong and courageous. Do not be frightened, and do not be dismayed, for the Lord your God is with you wherever you go." - Joshua 1:9 (ESV)

This would be the first thing I hung in his nursery. I knew this little boy inside of me would need a lot of strength to handle what was coming for him.

* * *

I had another ultrasound scheduled for nineteen weeks. I was feeling much better at that point and it looked like the nausea/vomiting was finally subsiding. We were also pleased to find out that the hyperthyroid medication was working. My thyroid levels were returning to normal.

I had to go alone to this appointment and was nervous about this ultrasound. This was around the point that we found out things weren't going well in Claire's pregnancy. I tried to stay calm and trust things would be different this time. As the ultrasound began, I held my breath. The sonographer moved the probe around on my belly and typed in some numbers. Then with a serious face, she said, "I'm so sorry Jenna, it looks like he is two weeks behind on his growth." My heart sunk.

I was taken to the examination room. I was sitting by myself in silence. The moment felt so surreal. I couldn't believe this was happening again. After all we had done to prepare, it was happening again.

The nurse walked in and took my vitals. My blood pressure had shot up to 170/110. My OBGYN then came in. He looked over his notes for a minute, then he solemnly said, "I am really sorry. It looks like you are developing preeclampsia. It is very rare for this to happen before twenty weeks and the outlook is not good." He explained that with all that was happening, it was going to be a challenge to get this pregnancy to twenty-four weeks. Twenty-four weeks is considered the "age of viability." This is the earliest in pregnancy that a fetus can survive outside of the womb. He told me to begin weekly appointments and said he would do all that he could.

I drove home from the appointment in silence. When I parked in the driveway, I stayed in my car and started to cry. "I can't handle what you're giving me," I cried. "I can't go through this again, I'm not strong enough. Please help me, God."

When I walked in, I told Mark the news. He held me in his arms as I cried. Twenty-four weeks seemed like an impossible hurdle to reach. Even if we made it to the "age of viability," what kind of life was this little boy going to have?

We were completely out of control and could do nothing but trust that this was out of our hands. We resolved that we would walk this road with open hands and love this little boy with all we had no matter what came.

* * *

I officially began bed rest at nineteen weeks. My blood pressure was okay in the mornings, so I tried to do a few fun things with Claire in the mornings around the house. Thankfully, she was still napping in the afternoons. That was when the preeclampsia would hit the hardest. My blood pressure would go from under 120/80 in the mornings and suddenly shoot up to 170/110 in the afternoons. When this would happen, I would get an intense, horrible headache. This would be followed by floating lightning bolts in my vision. I was so scared I would have a seizure.

My afternoons would be spent lying on my left side in bed with a blood pressure cuff strapped to my arm. I would lie there and pray that the baby and I would survive. I began to become obsessed with my blood pressure and was taking it several times an hour. I felt so out of control and was constantly entertaining the thought that I could die at any moment. All I could see was this giant mountain in front of me that I needed to climb. I was confident the feat would prove impossible.

The days were long, and the time dragged on very slowly. Our motto became, "choose joy" in our house. We couldn't control our circumstances, but we could control our attitudes. My sweet husband created a calendar with every possible holiday we could celebrate. Holidays such as Sandwich Day, Talk Like a Pirate Day, Pickle Day, Eat a Red Apple Day, Tongue Twister Day, and Caps Lock Day. Our texts to each other were very entertaining on Caps Lock Day.

We also had a big family party every Wednesday after my weekly check-ups to celebrate another week pregnant. We would get decorations and a cake. Claire loved it.

My family came in for about a week, to help with cooking, cleaning, and playing with Claire. They were a huge help to us during this time.

* * *

The big appointment finally came. I had made it to twenty-four weeks, the "age of viability." Mark and I both felt like we had just finished a marathon. We had reached the first big major hurtle and we were elated.

The ultrasound went well that day. Both the baby and I were doing well enough for us to continue the pregnancy. We had the biggest party we had ever had that afternoon.

We decided the time had come to give our baby boy a name. I had been putting it off because deep down I didn't know if he would survive. If we named him, I would just get more attached to him. But Mark was insistent that we give him a name.

We went back a fourth on some names for a few days, but neither of us really liked any of them. Suddenly, I thought about the name Drew, short for Andrew. Mark loved it. We looked up the meaning of the name, it meant, "strong and courageous." I looked at Mark, then looked at the sign I had hung in his room. It was the prayer I had been praying over this little baby since the beginning. There was no question, this little boy was meant to be named Andrew. We loved him with all we had.

* * *

We made it to our twenty-eight-week appointment. I never thought either us would have made it this far. The sonographer started the ultrasound. I knew the instant she started; it wasn't good. "He is now two and a half weeks behind on his growth and he is not moving the way we would like to see. His weight is 1 lb 12 oz. I am really sorry," she said kindly. My OBGYN said that we had done all we could do in the office and it was time for me to go to the hospital. He said to prepare to deliver him tomorrow.

I went home and was so frustrated. After all we did to prepare for this pregnancy, all we had gone through, and now this. Another one-pound preemie. Mark held me in his arms, then he took me to the hospital.

When I got to the hospital, they started me on magnesium through an IV to prepare for delivery. The magnesium would protect me from seizures and the baby from brain bleeds if I were to deliver the next day. I had an ultrasound with a specialist scheduled for the next day. My OBGYN wanted a second pair of eyes on the ultrasound before going through with delivery.

They kept me on magnesium overnight, and it was horrible. It makes your entire body feel like you are on fire. It caused my blood pressure to drop incredibly low and I almost lost consciousness. It caused extreme nausea and vomiting. I couldn't get out of bed because it caused my muscles to be extremely weak, so I had to use a bedpan. It was a miserable experience.

The next morning my OBGYN walked in with the MFM specialist. "Please take this IV out of my arm," I pleaded with him.

"I know the magnesium is awful," he said, "hang in there."

They performed the ultrasound. Drew wasn't doing great, but he was doing well enough to hold off with delivery. I would have to stay in the hospital and be monitored every three hours. They would also perform weekly ultrasounds to watch him closely.

Mark and Claire came to visit the next day on December 1, 2017. We kicked off the season of Advent in the hospital together. Mark brought an Advent calendar and we let Claire open a present. It was so heartbreaking to know how much of the holiday season I had missed with my little girl. Now I was going to have to miss even more. These were precious moments I would never get back and I was missing them.

They headed home and I was left alone in my hospital room. I was finally able to sit in silence and reflect on the reality of our situation. I couldn't believe it had turned out like this. Deep sadness and confusion washed over me. *Why couldn't my body work like it was supposed to? Why couldn't I do what every other woman could do? Why did this have to be so hard?*

* * *

The days in the hospital were spent similar to my days at home. I felt fairly good in the mornings and would be able to move around the room and sit up in a chair and read. Then the preeclampsia spells would hit in the afternoons. I brought my blood pressure cuff to the hospital and monitored it continuously, just like I did at home. The nurses seemed a little concerned I was so preoccupied with my blood pressure. They had never seen a patient bring their own blood pressure cuff into the hospital. But I didn't think anything of it. *It's just for right now*, I would reason to myself. *Once the pregnancy is over, I won't need to take it anymore.*

As time passed, being in the hospital got a little easier for me. It was a relief to now be in the care of knowledgeable, trustworthy nurses and doctors. Mark, on the other hand, was having to carry the full load back at home. He juggled working a full-time job with a boss that wasn't very sympathetic to our situation, taking care of our three-year-old, and handling all the household duties. He even made time every day for him and Claire to come to visit me. I was amazed by him. He did everything without complaining. He was our hero.

* * *

The days and weeks passed by slowly. The day came when I had made it to thirty-weeks and two days. I couldn't believe I had made it this long. I had been on bed rest with preeclampsia for almost three months at that point. Each week that passed with preeclampsia meant more time my baby boy wasn't getting enough oxygen and nutrients. I worried every day about what that was doing to him and how that would affect his development.

It was Friday, the day of my weekly ultrasound. The night before, I didn't sleep well. I felt horrible and wasn't feeling the baby kick as much as usual. In the morning, I woke up feeling a weird feeling in my head like I couldn't think straight.

The nurse walked in to take me to the ultrasound, and I said, "I think today's the day I'm going to deliver. My body can't do this anymore."

"Stay calm, let's see how the ultrasound goes," she said kindly.

My instinct was correct. As the specialist performed the ultrasound, his face became serious. He said that the amniotic fluid was extremely low, the baby was barely moving, and he was now three weeks behind on growth. It was time to take him out.

I called Mark and told him they were going to perform a c-section soon. His boss would not let him take off work, so I was going to have to go through this part alone.

A nurse brought me into a room. She hooked me back up to magnesium and prepped me for surgery. I was rolled into the operating room and was shaking uncontrollably. The doctors and nurses were so compassionate. One of the nurses offered to get my phone so she could take a picture of Drew after he was born. The NICU staff then came in and I felt immediate relief. It was as close to having family in there as I could get.

As they began the procedure, the anesthesiologist stayed by my head. He comforted me by saying, "You're doing great. Your blood pressure is good. Hang in there. They are almost done." He was the nicest doctor I had ever met.

Drew was born at 11:31am weighing 2 lb. 2 oz. The moment he came out of me I heard this sweet, high-pitched cry. My heart burst with love, and in that small moment, nothing else mattered. My baby was alive and crying. We had done it.

It was over.

* * *

I got to see my sweet baby very quickly after delivery, then they took him straight to the NICU. When I was being rolled out of the recovery room back to my hospital room, I saw Mark and Claire running towards me. Claire jumped into my arms. I held them both so tight. We had made it. The hardest part was finally over, and we could begin our journey back to normalcy.

* * *

The next morning, I was able to see Drew. They rolled my wheelchair up to his incubator, and all the memories of our first NICU journey came flooding back. Tears poured from my eyes. I didn't know if I had the strength to go through it all again. I put my hand over his incubator and prayed for another miracle.

* * *

Over the next few days, Drew was proving himself to be a very strong baby. He was nowhere near the "wimpy white boy," he was expected to be. They tried to put him on a ventilator when he was born, but he didn't need one. He was able to go directly to a CPAP after birth.

I was able to hold him just a few days after he was born, which was so special to me since I had to wait so long to hold Claire. The moment was just as meaningful. Drew and

I had been through so much together already. My heart burst with love for this courageous little boy.

I visited the NICU every day after Drew was born. Mark had some time off for the holidays, so I tried to spend as much time at the hospital as I could. I knew my visits would have to be much shorter once Mark went back to work because children under ten years old were not allowed in the NICU, so I wouldn't be able to bring Claire.

Drew had already transitioned off the CPAP and onto a nasal cannula a few days after he was born. It was looking as if our little boy had the same fight inside of him that his big sister had. I was so proud of our strong, little boy. It seemed that his NICU journey would be handled with ease.

I, on the other hand, was unknowingly about to face another battle of my own. Not a physical battle, but a battle in my mind.

Chapter Five

The Battle Rages On

It happened about a week after I got home from the hospital. I went to grab a shirt from my dresser drawer. As I reached into the drawer, I pulled out a t-shirt I had worn during my time on bed rest in the hospital. I stared at the red shirt and my heart started pounding, my face started sweating, and I began to shake. In an instant, I was back in the hospital. I could smell the hospital room and hear the sound of the monitor on my pregnant belly. It was as if I escaped reality for a moment. It was like my body was in my room, but my mind was back in the hospital.

Just as fast as it happened, I was back in reality and felt exhausted. I quickly grabbed every piece of clothing I had worn at the hospital. I threw all of them in the trash and tried to ignore what had just happened.

A few days later I was at the NICU visiting Drew. It was so much harder this time because I had Claire back at home to take care of. This meant I couldn't spend the same amount of time in the NICU with him as I did with Claire. That was so hard on me. I felt like I couldn't be a good mom to either of my children.

Drew was doing incredibly well. The doctors and nurses were impressed by his progress. He was completely off the nasal cannula after only a week in the NICU. He was able to breathe completely on his own. The only tube he had was a feeding tube in his nose. Basically, he was still there to grow and learn how to eat, then he could go home.

They had moved him into Claire's old room at the front of the NICU. It was a sweet gesture they did for us since we were NICU veterans. Everything was easier this time around. I felt more comfortable handling him and helping with baths and diaper changes. I was also able to take him out of his incubator on my own to hold him. He was doing well, which made this NICU stay far easier than the previous one.

After his "touch time" that day, I took him out of the incubator and placed him on my chest. I settled into the recliner next to the incubator for kangaroo care time. The nurse left me the call light and I settled in with my little boy.

Suddenly, my heart started pounding again. This time I was sure it was going to pound out of my chest. I started sweating and shaking. I was back in that hospital room again. I had a break from reality and was so scared something was going to happen to this tiny baby in my arms. I could smell all the smells and hear all the sounds in that room. I could feel a blood pressure cuff around my right arm.

I came back to reality quickly and had this sudden urge to run away. I took ten deep breaths and tried to calm myself down. I almost called the nurse, but I was afraid of what she might think. I managed to calm myself down and decided I couldn't tell anyone about this. I was so worried they would think I was crazy. I began to wonder if I really was going crazy.

* * *

Over the next few weeks, I visited the NICU as often as possible, all while trying to juggle taking care of my now four-year-old and healing from my c-section. My blood pressure was not going down as it did with my first pregnancy. I went on to find out that the prolonged preeclampsia my body endured caused irreversible damage to my kidneys. I would need to see a nephrologist every year, and I would need to be on a small dose of blood pressure medication, possibly for the rest of my life.

Drew was doing amazingly well in the NICU. He was growing and was now in an open crib. He first tried taking a bottle at thirty-two weeks gestation, and he took to it instantly. He had taken an entire bottle on his third try, the nurses were amazed. He, thankfully, wasn't having any apnea episodes while trying to eat. He even cried when he was hungry. The nurse told me he was the only preemie that young she had ever seen cry for food. We later went on to nickname him, "The Food Dude." He absolutely loved to eat. I felt so blessed to have two preemies who were good eaters. The chances of having that happen were extremely low.

I was still silently dealing with the "break from reality" episodes. They came on randomly and out of nowhere. I had also developed extreme anxiety. I felt that at any moment something was going to happen to me. Every morning I woke up wondering if I would die that day. It was all I could do to keep it together on the outside, but on the inside, I was a wreck.

* * *

The day came on Sunday, January 21, 2018. As I walked into the NICU that afternoon, one of Drew's nurses came over to me. She said, "You might need to sit down for this." I went into Drew's room, and she said, "Well, I know Drew has only been here for five weeks, and I know he is still extremely small. But he is doing so well we just cannot keep him here anymore. He's going to be discharged on Tuesday."

I was in shock. I barely had time to recover from my surgery, and I was just beginning to process what had happened in the past five months. I had expected he would be in the NICU until around his due date, which was February 21, 2018. Now we were expected to bring home a baby who was thirty-five weeks gestation. He wasn't even supposed to be born for five more weeks. I suddenly felt extremely overwhelmed.

The next day the nurse walked me through all the discharge information. There was much less to have to deal with than there was the first time around since we didn't have to deal with oxygen and a monitor.

After explaining all the discharge information, the nurse asked me how I was doing. I nonchalantly said, "I've been having a little anxiety, but it's probably just the hormones." She said that it was common to feel that way after all I went through and to tell my doctor if it continues more than two months.

That afternoon, Mark, Claire, and I loaded our 3 lb. 8 oz. baby into his car seat and headed home as a family of four.

* * *

Drew showed himself to be a very calm, content baby after bringing him home from the hospital. He slept peacefully in his swing or the Moby Wrap most of the day, only to wake for feedings. He would get a little fussy in the evenings, but it didn't last nearly as long as it did with Claire. Everything was much easier this time around.

He was so incredibly tiny, about as long as our forearms. He was as cute as he could be, and Claire absolutely loved being his big sister. She would rock him in his swing singing, "Rudolph the Red Nose Reindeer" as he slept quietly. She loved helping us give him baths and encouraged him during tummy time. She was such a patient, loving, and kind older sister. We were amazed at how little jealousy she had towards him and how quickly she stepped up into her role as the oldest sibling.

Mark and I had a much easier time this time around. Four years of marriage helped us to learn how to deal with stress and conflict in a much healthier way. We were able to tackle having two kids as a strong team.

Drew hit all his milestones right on time just like his big sister. We were so amazed and grateful that after all he had been through, he was developing just like any other baby. He was living up to his name and impressing everyone.

It was such a blessing that Drew was an easier infant than Claire because it wasn't until after we brought him home from the NICU that my battle really began.

* * *

When I was on bed rest during the pregnancy, I was anticipating the day that I wouldn't have to worry about my blood pressure anymore. I assumed that after delivery I would put the blood pressure machine away in the closet and move on with my life.

Unfortunately, I didn't consider how my mind was being trained. I had formed an obsession, and obsessions don't easily go away. I thought about my blood pressure 24/7. Even though I was able to resist taking it more than a couple of times a day after the pregnancy, my mind was constantly fixated on it. I was always wondering whether it was high or low. I was constantly worried that it would spike up without me knowing, and I would have a seizure or a stroke. I would talk to Mark daily about what everyone should do if something were to happen to me.

I also was in a constant state of alertness. I could never calm down and relax. Every sound I heard caused me to jump. I could hardly ever sit down. If I did, I had to have music or the TV on in the background, something to distract me from the anxiety. That anxiety caused me to be irritable and easily agitated. I tried my best not to act out of my agitation, but occasionally I would find myself snap out of nowhere. I was not myself and it was starting to affect the ones I loved the most.

One night I couldn't sleep, so I started to browse the internet to try to figure out what was going on with me. My OBGYN had said that postpartum anxiety was normal for the first month or so after pregnancy. I googled, "postpartum anxiety," but the symptoms just didn't really fit with what I was experiencing.

I decided instead to just type in the symptoms I was experiencing and see what came up. The instant I hit the "search" button, it popped up everywhere: Post Traumatic Stress Disorder (PTSD). I scrolled through all the symptoms: hypervigilance, catastrophizing, flashbacks, nightmares, agitation, exaggerated startle response. It all fit. I knew for certain that was what I was experiencing.

I spent the next hour watching YouTube videos that addressed PTSD. I found a wonderful therapist who put out several videos about PTSD and did a great job of explaining what it was.

She said that PTSD has a lot to do with the formation of memories. Our brain can form two different types of memories, non-traumatic memories, and traumatic memories. Non-traumatic memories are the memories your brain prefers. They are safe and predictable. For example, say you go to the beach with a friend one day. You drive down, eat at a restaurant overlooking the water, spend some time in the sand, then come home. Your brain is easily able to process that event. Nothing out of the ordinary or threatening happened, and it's all in a nice, predictable order. It puts that memory in a nice filing folder labeled, "My Day at the Beach," and puts it in a filing cabinet. When you need to recall the event, your brain can easily access it and retrieve your memory of that day.

Traumatic memories are handled differently. Traumatic memories are memories that are created when something so fearful, so uncontrollable, and so overwhelming happens that our brains cannot process it. It's as if these memories get frantically written down, and instead of getting put into a file, they just get thrown all over our filing cabinet. There's no way for our brain to make sense of the traumatic event, so it just becomes a big mess of unorganized memories. Your brain tries to bring up these memories to process them, and when this happens, it's called a "flashback." The "break from reality" events I was experiencing finally made sense to me.

She then went on to explain the other symptoms characterizing PTSD. She did this by discussing two parts of the brain: the amygdala and the prefrontal cortex. These brain structures physically change with PTSD. The amygdala, which is the part of the brain that is responsible for the "fight or flight" response gets bigger. The prefrontal cortex, which is responsible for rational, critical thinking gets smaller. So, your amygdala begins to take over your brain, so to speak. This results in a constant state of "fight or flight." And with a smaller prefrontal cortex, you're less able to produce rational thoughts. The good news was that with proper treatment, MRI scans have shown that these two brain regions will return to their proper size.

I felt empowered by this information. I considered seeking out treatment, but I was too worried about what people would think. I concluded that now that I understood what was going on in my brain, I would be able to control it. I felt confident that with enough willpower I could overcome this.

* * *

As much as I thought I could control the PTSD, it got worse and worse as time went on. The flashbacks became more frequent and more severe.

One Saturday morning, I decided Claire and I should go have a little Mommy/Daughter time together. I asked her what she wanted to do, and without hesitation, she said, "Let's go to Old West Cafe!" Old West Cafe was a local breakfast place, that we would argue makes the best food in Texas. We headed out excited for some good food and good conversation.

The moment I walked into the restaurant, a flashback hit hard. We had come to that restaurant several times when I was experiencing hyperemesis gravidarum. I was never able to eat anything because I was so sick, but I wanted to come along for the company. Some smell must have triggered those memories because suddenly I felt incredibly nauseated. My head was sweating and my heart pounding. I tried to play it off and pretend like I was fine. I smiled and laughed with Claire during our meal, all the while I felt like I was going to explode inside with angst and panic. The flashback lasted until our meal was over and we left the restaurant. I knew I could never go back there again.

Another day, I had put Drew down for a nap and Claire was coloring at the dining room table. It was raining outside, and the humidity was rising. I looked at our thermostat and the humidity read ninety-six percent. The number ninety-six threw me into another flashback. Suddenly I was sitting on the couch with the blood pressure cuff strapped around my arm and the machine in my lap. The reading was 160/96. Panic flooded my body. I came back to reality and had to get down on my knees to try to calm myself down.

"What's wrong Mommy?" Claire asked from the table.

"Oh, I'm okay. Don't worry. Mommy's fine!" But I knew I wasn't fine. I had to do something about this.

I finally shared what I was going through with Mark, who, thankfully, didn't think I was crazy. I had concluded that the only logical thing to do was to sell our house and move. *If I could escape all the things that trigger my flashbacks, then I'll be fine*, I thought.

Mark agreed. He would do anything to help. He was just as convinced as I was that moving would take away my flashbacks.

We quickly put our house on the market and found another house in a town only about twenty minutes away. We packed our bags and I said goodbye to the house that was full of so many horrible memories.

* * *

The distractions that come with moving with a four-year-old and a three-month-old were greatly beneficial for me. I was so wrapped up in packing, unpacking, and decorating, that my symptoms of PTSD subsided substantially. I thought that our plan was working, and I would be free of this horrible mental illness.

Unfortunately, it was a momentary success. After a few weeks, once we were settled into our new home, the symptoms came back with a vengeance. The flashbacks were the worst offenders. I began having flashbacks of my flashbacks, and they were occurring multiple times a day. I was also more on edge than I had ever been. I never felt calm. I was a wreck.

One sunny morning in August, I decided to take the kids for a walk. I loaded the baby into the stroller, and we set out for a walking path near our new home.

As we were walking on the path, I realized we were completely alone. I started to panic. I had visions of a rabid dog jumping out from the trees to attack us. I worried that a man would jump out from the bushes and take Claire. I kept telling Claire to stay close to me and asked her to hold my hand throughout the entire walk.

When we got home, I started to cry. I couldn't do this anymore. Something was seriously wrong, and I couldn't handle it on my own. I needed help.

I looked up counselors near me and called the first place on the list. It turned out this counselor not only happened to specialize in trauma, but pregnancy-related trauma. And her office was five minutes from our house.

I made my first appointment and prayed that this counselor would free me from the battle in my mind.

Chapter Six

Healing

The day of my first therapy appointment arrived. I was anxious but also hopeful to find healing. Mark was working from home, so I was able to schedule my appointments during Drew's afternoon nap. I put Drew down, gave Mark the baby monitor, and headed to the counselor's office.

After arriving, I waited in the waiting room for about ten minutes, I found myself feeling extremely uncomfortable. Everyone in that waiting room knew every other person was struggling with a mental illness. It was hard to be put in a category that has such a social stigma in our society.

"Jenna?" a woman said as she opened the door. I got up and followed her into the back room.

She introduced herself and we got down to business. I told her all that I had been struggling with and she confirmed a diagnosis of PTSD. She said that there was a treatment that was starting to get a lot of attention. It started out with a lot of push-back from the counseling community. But as research began to come out to support it, professionals began to give it more respect. It was called Eye Movement Desensitization and Reprocessing (EMDR). She explained that EMDR was based on the knowledge that the processing of memories occurs during rapid eye movement (REM) sleep. If we could mimic REM sleep while we were awake, our brains would be able to process traumatic events in a controlled environment.

During EMDR, REM sleep was mimicked by bilateral stimulation of the brain using eye movements. I wasn't going to be in a hypnotic state. I would, however, feel like I was dreaming.

We spent the rest of our first session getting a plan established and figuring out the best way for me to go through the EMDR treatment. I tried the eye movements, but it was too distracting, so we used pulsars in my hands instead. I held one pulsar in each hand. When she turned on the machine, I would feel a pulse in one hand, then the other. This bilateral pulsation would put my brain in a state that would allow it to process my traumatic memories.

I was a bit skeptical of the treatment. She reassured me that the research was promising, and she had seen it work very well with her patients. I decided that it was worth a try.

She told me that we would start the treatment at the next week's appointment. We would do as many appointments as it took for me to be completely back to my old self. I made an appointment for the next week and headed home.

The first thing we did at my next appointment was to establish a "safe space" in my mind. It was a place I could retreat to if I became too anxious. I felt a little weird doing this. The whole experience of therapy was very foreign to me, and it was way out of my comfort zone. But I went ahead and went forward with it. I was willing to try anything at that point.

The place I chose was my college dorm room. Freshman year of college gave me all the freedom of being an adult, with almost none of the responsibility. It was the freest I have ever felt in my life. In that dorm room, I was shielded from the difficulty and dangers of the real world. I was safe.

Then we began EMDR. She turned on the pulsars and I closed my eyes. She told me to go to my "safe space" and to rate my anxiety on a scale from 0-10. I told her it was zero, so we went to the next step. She told me to close my eyes and recall a scary, traumatic moment during my pregnancy. The image that popped into my mind was sitting in the truck outside of the Old West Café. Many times we would wait in the car while we waited for our table to be ready. The smell of bacon and pancakes filled the air. Claire was in the back of the truck watching a show on the iPad. The sound of that show mixed with the smell in the air triggered me to feel nauseated and panicked. I began to sweat.

The therapist stopped me and gave me a list of phrases that described how I felt. I chose the phrase, "I'm out of control, I cannot handle this." Then she told me to choose a phrase I wanted to believe about this event. I chose the phrase, "It's over, I'm safe now."

She then told me to rate my anxiety from 0-10. I told her it was ten. She told me to close my eyes and let my brain try to process this event. I closed my eyes and suddenly felt as if I was dreaming. Nothing really makes a lot of sense in a dream. There were a lot of random things that came in and out of my mind, just like I was dreaming. She would occasionally stop me to see how my anxiety was doing, then I would go back into it. Toward the end of my "dream," I was back sitting in the front seat of the truck outside the restaurant. I looked down at my belly and suddenly I wasn't pregnant anymore. I turned around and looked in the backseat. Drew was sitting peacefully in his car seat and Claire was happily watching her show. My nausea was gone. I felt normal again. I said to myself, "It's over, I'm safe now." I then had a peace wash over me. We all got out of the car and went into the restaurant to eat.

I opened my eyes and told the therapist that my anxiety was now at a zero. She had me close my eyes and end the session in my "safe space."

The goal of every EMDR session was to end the session with an anxiety rating close to zero. Therefore, it was a success. As we were finishing up the session, she told me that it was common for my PTSD symptoms to get worse before they get better. But she wanted me to push through it since she was certain I was on the road to healing.

* * *

The next few months rolled by. Claire started Pre-K, and I got to spend the days with my sweet little guy. He was now close to getting through his first year of life. He was a sweet, chatty baby with a loud, contagious laugh. He absolutely loved his mommy and was just as much of a "Velcro Baby" as his big sister was. He was such a happy baby. Claire gave him the nickname, "Smiley Guyly." He loved being around other kids. Thankfully, because his NICU stay was much easier than Claire's was, we didn't have to be as intense with lock-down this time around. We got to go to parks, the library, and play dates with friends.

He was continuing to develop right on track and didn't need any intervention. I was watching another prayer being answered and another miracle evolve before my very eyes.

The weekly therapy sessions were helping tremendously. I was very surprised; I didn't expect it to help so much. During my sessions, I was working through different memories of the pregnancy and delivery each week. Each time I came up with a new phrase my mind needed to accept before it could process the memory. Then we would work through EMDR until I believed that phrase and my anxiety was rated a zero. My PTSD symptoms were variable after the therapy sessions. They were usually good for a few days after the sessions and then got worse as the week went on.

The day came when I experienced a major breakthrough. It was Halloween. Claire and Drew were dressed as Violet and Jack-Jack from The Incredibles. They were so adorable. We planned to eat pizza for dinner, then go out trick-or-treating in our new neighborhood. Our old neighborhood was mostly full of older couples without kids. Our new neighborhood constantly looked like someone had kicked a kid ant hill. We were so excited to get a real trick-or-treating experience.

My anxiety was high that day from the moment I woke up and I didn't know why. I also dealt with several flashbacks throughout the day, which was a rare thing at that point. I was feeling so disheartened. It seemed like all the progress I was making the past few months was being wiped away.

I made it through the day and enjoyed trick-or-treating with my sweet family. After trick-or-treating, I went upstairs to put Drew down to sleep. He loved for me to rock him in his rocking chair in the dark before putting him down to sleep. Suddenly, as I was rocking Drew in the rocking chair, flashbacks and anxiety hit like a tidal wave. It was as if my mind was replaying every single event from the time I got pregnant to the time I delivered. This went on for about two or three minutes. Then, in an instant, it was over. All my anxiety and all my fears were gone just like that. It was as if a huge weight was suddenly lifted off my shoulders. I felt like I was myself again, the way I felt before the pregnancy. I hadn't felt like that in such a long time. It was as if my mind went through major processing of all my traumatic events in one moment, and then it was finished.

Over the next week, I felt incredibly better. I still had a flashback here and there, but they were far less severe. I was so eager to tell my therapist about what had happened.

During the next session, I shared my breakthrough with my therapist, and she was astonished. She said the success of EMDR never ceased to amaze her. She said that because I was still experiencing flashbacks, there must be one more thing that my brain needed to process through. Once I could target that thing, I would be completely healed. She asked me to go through the list of phrases and see if there was a phrase that I still didn't believe. I scrolled the list and my eyes instantly stopped at the phrase, "I'm okay." Through this whole ordeal, my biggest struggle was believing that I was strong, that my body wouldn't fail me. I felt fragile. I knew this was the last and most difficult thing I was going to need to believe.

We started the session. I entered into my dream state. I was sitting on the couch in our old house with my blood pressure cuff strapped to my arm. The machine was showing an exceedingly high reading. I sat there not knowing what to do. I felt lost and out of control. Just then, I saw a folder appear on the kitchen table. I walked over and grabbed the folder. I walked back to the couch and opened it. It was the results of a medical scan with my name on it. I spent time going through all the results, and they revealed that I was completely healthy. I had no health issues whatsoever. Suddenly, I looked up. The house was packed up with boxes. "Are you coming?" Mark called from outside the front door. I stood up and walked to the door. I looked back one last time. Everything was packed away and gone. The sun was shining brightly through the windows, and the house was bright and clean. Everything looked new and beautiful. "I'm okay," I whispered to myself. Then I closed the door and left.

As I was driving home from my final therapy session, I saw the fall leaves blow across the road. I thought about my amazing husband and two precious kids I was driving home to and all we had survived together. I looked forward to all the things we were about to celebrate in the coming weeks. I remembered all that we had been through, and how far we had come. I thought about all the things we had to look forward to in the future. Gratefulness and peace covered me like a warm blanket.

I took a big, deep breath in and out and whispered confidently to myself, "I'm okay."

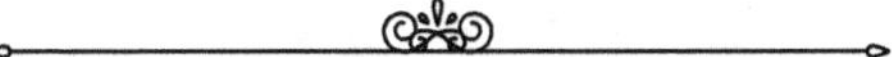

PART TWO

THE LESSON

Chapter Seven

Guilt

The first moments I saw my tiny babies, surrounded with tubes and machines, fighting for their lives, all I could say to them, through tear-filled eyes was, "I'm sorry." *I'm sorry that I couldn't protect you like I was supposed to. I'm sorry that my body failed you. I'm sorry that you're having to experience all this suffering and you are struggling to stay alive, while most babies your age are safe and content inside their mother's wombs.*

My OBGYN said something I didn't expect after my first delivery. The surgery was finished, and Claire was being transported to the NICU. My doctor told the nurses to wait to administer the morphine. He said he had something to tell me that was important for me to remember. He patted me on the arm, looked at me, and said, "You did everything you could have done. You did everything right. This was not your fault."

As I was standing over my tiny baby lying in her incubator the next day, watching her little lungs laboring to breathe, I heard those words from my doctor, "This was not your fault." He knew the words I needed to hear, and I held onto them. He had been doing this long enough to know that guilt would be the initial emotion a woman would experience after a premature delivery.

I desperately wanted to believe that our situation was not my fault. I would hear preachers say that God is in control of everything and everything happens for a reason, but it was so difficult to let that truth settle into my heart. I could never seem to stop thinking about what I could have done differently during the pregnancies. I couldn't help but think the outcome could have changed if I had done something different. I couldn't handle the idea that I might have done something to cause the suffering that my babies had to endure.

I struggled with guilt differently after both pregnancies. After my first pregnancy, I wondered if I should've stopped working right away when I found out I was pregnant. The hospital is an incredibly stressful work environment. I was sure I would have been able to go longer in the pregnancy if I had not been so stressed out. I wondered if I should've taken the doctors more seriously and heeded their wisdom. I was so proud and naive. *Who was I to think I knew better than specialists who had been doing nothing but working with pregnant women for thirty years?* I wondered if traveling on a plane at twenty-three weeks pregnant made things worse. I shudder to think about what my blood pressure reading was on the plane when I felt so horrible. I even thought about the little things, like that one time I accidentally ate feta on my salad or lifted too much weight at the gym. I feared every little thing might have contributed to her difficult beginning and her possible future difficulties.

It didn't help that I had well-meaning people say things to me after Claire's pregnancy that were so unhelpful. Some said that medical doctors were incompetent. They would say that my OBGYN only knew how to perform surgery, so when things began to go wrong in the pregnancy, it was the only action he knew how to take. They would say these things without taking the time to research his expertise and experience. They quickly blamed him without knowing anything about the situation.

Those same people would tell me that if I had just done certain things that this never would have happened. Things like eating organic foods, taking certain supplements, using essential oils, and seeing an alternative medicine practitioner instead of a medical doctor.

I knew cognitively that these things weren't true. I had known enough women who had done none of those things and had perfectly healthy pregnancies and natural labor and deliveries. I also really trusted my OBGYN. He was such a caring, compassionate, and competent doctor. In my mind, he was the one who saved both of our lives.

Although I knew these things were untrue, the comments still stung. It felt as if I was being blamed for what happened in my pregnancy. I was confident that I would have done absolutely anything to protect my baby and create a better outcome for her. Hearing comments like these only increased the guilt I felt. I was already blaming myself. Now other people were blaming me as well.

During my second pregnancy, I struggled with a whole new kind of guilt. I still felt the same things I did after my first pregnancy, but with some additions. Mainly, I wondered if I was blinded by my own ambition and didn't assess the risks seriously enough before getting pregnant. I wanted another baby so badly, and the achiever in me had a strong desire for a do-over. I was so sure I could do it. I knew several women who went on to have full-term babies after a premature delivery. I was certain that my body could work like every other woman's body did if I just got another chance. But when I stood over my two-pound baby boy in an incubator and realized I had failed again, I feared what the future held. I certainly didn't regret having him, I loved him deeply and was so incredibly grateful for him. But the prognosis was bleak, and I was responsible for bringing this little guy into the world where he may struggle significantly. I wondered if I had brought him into the world just for him to suffer.

At my four-week follow-up after my second pregnancy, I brought up my feelings of guilt with my OBGYN. I spoke to him specifically about my fear that I had done something to cause the outcomes of my pregnancies. He reassured me saying, "It's very normal for a woman to feel guilty when something goes wrong in her pregnancy. I have seen women do everything wrong in pregnancy and have healthy, full-term deliveries. Then I have seen, as in your case, women who do everything right, and have everything go wrong. You did all you could to have a healthy pregnancy. Sometimes things just happen in pregnancy that are out of our control."

I was able to reason that we did all we could with the information we were given during both pregnancies. I would have done absolutely anything to keep my baby safe inside of me, but you don't know what you don't know. We did all that we could and all we could do is move forward with the future in mind. However, even with my resolve, that pesky guilt would creep back up on me for years to follow.

There were many times I would look at my babies and wonder how their lives would be different had they not been so premature. *Would they be more confident? Would they have more friends? Would school be easier for them? Would they not be left out when trying to play with their much larger peers?* Then I would remember how good we had it. Both Claire and Drew made it out of their NICU journeys largely unscathed. That's not the case with so many premature babies. Remembering this would cause me to feel guilty for worrying about things that seemed insignificant when compared to what other preemie parents were dealing with.

Guilt became my closest companion, and it was keeping me in a cage of self-pity and paralyzing me from moving forward. Guilt is an interesting emotion. There is guilt caused by something you did to hurt another person, in which you are definitely in the wrong. But there's another kind of guilt. A guilt that is unwarranted. A type of guilt that you put on yourself, even though there is no proof that you did anything wrong. Either way, guilt is like a cancer of the soul. It sits waiting for the right time to strike, then attacks unrelentingly. It steals your joy and freedom in an instant.

Best-selling novelist, Sabaa Tahir once said, "There are two kinds of guilt: the kind that drowns you until you're useless, and the kind that fires your soul to purpose." I couldn't change the past. I couldn't go back and undo what had happened. If I let guilt overtake my life, I would be rendered useless.

I had two choices. I could sit in my guilt and despair, or I could use my circumstances to push me forward to a greater meaning and purpose. But I couldn't shake the difficulty I had with suffering, why bad things happened to good people. I couldn't move forward without answering some difficult questions. *Why would a loving God allow pain into our lives? Could there be a greater purpose for our suffering?*

Chapter Eight

Why Me, God?

There is a type of theology that exists in the Christian world, called the *Prosperity Gospel*, that teaches if you are a true believer and have a strong enough faith, God will give you health, wealth, and prosperity.

Leaders of this movement use certain Bible verses to support their claim:

> *"For truly, I say to you, if you have faith like a grain of mustard seed, you will say to this mountain, 'Move from here to there,' and it will move, and nothing will be impossible for you." Matthew 17:20b (ESV)*

> *"For I know the plans I have for you," declares the Lord, "plans to prosper you and not to harm you, plans to give you hope and a future." Jeremiah 29:11 (NIV)*

"For you know the grace of our Lord Jesus Christ, that though he was rich, yet for your sake he became poor, so that you through his poverty might become rich." 2 Corinthians 8:9 (ESV)

I never really knew much about this theology when I was young. I grew up in a home of non-Christians. When I was ten years old my best friend invited me to a church camp. It was there that I heard the message of the Gospel for the first time and became a follower of Christ. Growing up, I was taught that God loved us and was in control of everything in our lives. Christians and non-Christians alike will encounter suffering in this life because we live in a broken world, but there will be a day when Christ returns and abolishes evil and suffering for good.

It wasn't until my late twenties that I was introduced to the prosperity theology. There is something so alluring about health, wealth, and prosperity. Being able to have control over my life was something the "type A" in me loved. *All I have to do is have faith and God will give me what I want? Sounds good to me!* I thought.

After my first pregnancy went wrong, I concluded that the suffering we endured was caused by my lack of faith. When I found out I was pregnant again, my faith was strong and confident. I prayed "expectantly" just like I was supposed to do. I was certain that God would answer my prayer for a healthy, full-term pregnancy.

When things started going wrong, my faith was hit hard. I couldn't understand why God wasn't answering my prayer. It was a good prayer. I wanted good for my baby. I wanted our story to be redeemed. That's how I wanted God to show his power and goodness, by giving us good things. *Was he punishing me? Was my faith not strong enough?* These doubts and questions turned into confusion and disappointment and an eventual turning away from God. For months after Drew was born, I couldn't pray, I couldn't read my Bible, I even questioned whether God was real.

I fell into a deep well of resentment and sadness. I would see women with their big pregnant bellies and feel so hurt and confused. *Why did they get it so easy when I had it so hard? Why me, God? Why did this happen to me?* The ugliness of my heart really came out when I found out the woman wasn't a Christian. *She doesn't even love God and everything is so easy for her. She gets an easy pregnancy and perfect full-term baby with no effort at all. I faithfully served God for so many years and this is how He repays me.*

Over those months, although the sinfulness of my heart had taken over, I still felt God's presence. He never left me. His steadfast love sustained me. These verses proved themselves true in my life:

"I give them eternal life, and they will never perish, and no one will snatch them out of my hand." John 10:28 (ESV)

"For I am sure that neither death nor life, nor angels nor rulers, nor things present nor things to come, nor powers, nor height nor depth, nor anything else in all creation, will be able to separate us from the love of God in Christ Jesus our Lord." Romans 8:38-39 (ESV)

During those months following my pregnancy with Drew, I began diving into apologetics. I had never objectively studied Christianity, and I was at a point where I felt I needed to find the evidence for my faith. Over my time of studying, I found that the evidence for Jesus' life and resurrection was just too strong to deny. If He was who He said He was, then the Bible was trustworthy. I may not like how God chose to handle things in my life, but who was I to question the One who created this universe.

One day I sat down and read my Bible again. I opened it to this story:

"And he said, "There was a man who had two sons. And the younger of them said to his father, 'Father, give me the share of property that is coming to me.' And he divided his property between them. Not many days later, the younger son gathered all he had and took a journey into a far country, and there he squandered

his property in reckless living. And when he had spent everything, a severe famine arose in that country, and he began to be in need. So he went and hired himself out to one of the citizens of that country, who sent him into his fields to feed pigs. And he was longing to be fed with the pods that the pigs ate, and no one gave him anything.

"But when he came to himself, he said, 'How many of my father's hired servants have more than enough bread, but I perish here with hunger! I will arise and go to my father, and I will say to him, "Father, I have sinned against heaven and before you. I am no longer worthy to be called your son. Treat me as one of your hired servants."' And he arose and came to his father. But while he was still a long way off, his father saw him and felt compassion, and ran and embraced him and kissed him. And the son said to him, 'Father, I have sinned against heaven and before you. I am no longer worthy to be called your son.' But the father said to his servants, 'Bring quickly the best robe, and put it on him, and put a ring on his hand, and shoes on his feet. And bring the fattened calf and kill it, and let us eat and celebrate. For this my son was dead, and is alive again; he was lost, and is found.' And they began to celebrate.

"Now his older son was in the field, and as he came and drew near to the house, he heard music and dancing.

And he called one of the servants and asked what these things meant. And he said to him, 'Your brother has come, and your father has killed the fattened calf, because he has received him back safe and sound.' But he was angry and refused to go in. His father came out and entreated him, but he answered his father, 'Look, these many years I have served you, and I never disobeyed your command, yet you never gave me a young goat, that I might celebrate with my friends. But when this son of yours came, who has devoured your property with prostitutes, you killed the fattened calf for him!' And he said to him, 'Son, you are always with me, and all that is mine is yours. It was fitting to celebrate and be glad, for this your brother was dead, and is alive; he was lost, and is found.'" Luke 15:11–32 (ESV)

As I was reading this story, I quickly began to resonate with the prodigal son. But then God revealed something to me. I thought I resembled the prodigal son, but in reality, I far more resembled the older brother. I hadn't really run away from God. I was the one stubbornly sitting in my pride and resentment for not getting what I felt I deserved. I was angry at God because I felt I deserved something from him from all those years of faithfully following him. When I saw other people getting what I felt I deserved, I pridefully concluded that I should be getting the good things they were given. This parable clearly revealed to me that my view of God was wrong. We do not earn His love and goodness with our good works. He freely gives His love and mercy to all people. We do not follow His commands to get something from Him, we obey Him because He is a father who knows what is best for us. His commands always lead us to joy. It always gets us more of Him.

My heart was full of destructive pride that God was slowly working out of me. I didn't want to be the person I had become. I knelt down, repented, and asked for forgiveness. I immediately felt God's mercy and forgiveness wash over me. My eyes were opened, and my heart was humbled.

* * *

After turning back to the Lord, I began to study more about the theology that had failed me. The reason *The Prosperity Gospel* is so appealing is that it promises to give us our idols. But when we chase idols, we will ultimately be disappointed, because idols are fleeting and do not give lasting satisfaction.

For me, a healthy pregnancy and healthy, full-term baby became my idol. I thought that if I just got it, I would be happy. My life would be complete.

Idols promise to give us what only God can give, lasting comfort and eternal satisfaction. But they cannot fulfill that promise. They give us momentary fulfillment and satisfaction, but it never lasts. It's like building the foundation of your house on sand rather than concrete. Everything is great if circumstances around the house are good, but once a storm hits, the house is quickly brought down to the ground.

The *Prosperity Gospel* sounds so appealing. Nobody wants to suffer, and I'm not sure I know anyone who would not sign up for a pain-free life. But the *Prosperity Gospel* has missed the mark. God does want us to prosper, just not in the way the *Prosperity Gospel* would teach. He wants us to have deep, lasting joy that is independent of circumstances. This kind of joy is found in living for God, rather than ourselves. It is only when our life is focused on the advancement of The Kingdom that our joy will be complete. When the Bible speaks of riches and prosperity, it is almost never referring to worldly riches, but spiritual riches.

Paul Tripp, a well-known Bible teacher once said:

"When God prospers people who are no longer living for their own selfish desires but are living for His will, the result is the furtherance of His kingdom purposes on earth, which results in His glory....So, is it right to pray for prosperity? It is and you should. Not for the sake of your kingdom, but for the success of His."

The irony of the *Prosperity Gospel* is that it leads people away from what will actually prosper them. It is only when we fully surrender our lives to God with open hands, accepting anything he allows into our lives, that we will experience true prosperity.

Throughout this journey of healing physically, mentally, and spiritually, I stopped asking the question, "Why me, God?" I came to accept that His ways are far beyond my understanding. I am part of a bigger story and I am not the main character. All the events that occur in my life are meant to glorify God and point others to Him. It is through those events that I will obtain more joy, freedom, and maturity. And sometimes the only way this occurs is through suffering.

Chapter Nine

Count it All Joy

There is one main thing I have learned from our season of difficulty and struggle. It is that contrary to common belief, suffering is not God's wrath and anger on a believer's life. When we suffer, we are not being punished for not having enough faith. I have come to find that suffering is actually God's grace in our lives.

Suffering is a major theme in the Bible, from the Old Testament through the New Testament. It would seem that God allows us to suffer for various reasons. It may be to reveal His sovereignty to His people or to work in us the process of sanctification. Sometimes the reason we suffer is simply the fact that we are living in a broken world. A world in which suffering naturally occurs.

One of the first stories in the Bible that we learn of God's hand in our suffering is from the book of Job:

"There was a man in the land of Uz whose name was Job, and that man was blameless and upright, one who feared God and turned away from evil...Now there was a day when the sons of God came to present themselves before the LORD, and Satan also came among them. The LORD said to Satan, "From where have you come?" Satan answered the LORD and said, "From going to and fro on the earth, and from walking up and down on it." And the LORD said to Satan, "Have you considered my servant Job, that there is none like him on the earth, a blameless and upright man, who fears God and turns away from evil?" Then Satan answered the LORD and said, "Does Job fear God for no reason? Have you not put a hedge around him and his house and all that he has, on every side? You have blessed the work of his hands, and his possessions have increased in the land. But stretch out your hand and touch all that he has, and he will curse you to your face." And the LORD said to Satan, "Behold, all that he has is in your hand. Only against him do not stretch out your hand." So Satan went out from the presence of the LORD." Job 1:1-12 (ESV)

There are two things to take away from these first twelve verses. First, God is in complete control of everything in the universe, including evil. Satan was unable to do anything to Job, without first asking God's permission. And God set perimeters in which he was able to act.

The second take-away from these verses is that our righteousness and strong faith does not guarantee we will experience a life free from suffering. This was a hard truth I had to learn for myself after my second pregnancy. Job was "blameless and upright," but that did not stop the suffering that was going to come into his life.

Paul Tripp summarized the book of Job in the following way:

"Do we achieve the favor of God, the blessings of God, by means of our performance? The devastating answer of Job is, 'Absolutely not,' because human righteousness always falls short of God's standard. And so, Job destroys and decimates human understanding of what's fair...You would read Job and say it's not fair for Job to suffer. On what standard? No one deserves God's favor. No one deserves His blessing. The most righteous person you could name falls short. That's the penetrating drama of Job."

The entire meta-narrative of the Bible is that humankind is not able, no matter how hard they try, to live up to God's standards. This is the reason Jesus needed to come. He lived a perfect life then suffered and died for us. Through this, he imparted His perfect life to us and absorbed the punishment that was meant for us. If we believe this message, we should know wholeheartedly that our good works in life do not win us right standing with God.

The book of Job continues, and unfortunately for Job, things get worse:

"Now there was a day when his sons and daughters were eating and drinking wine in their oldest brother's house, and there came a messenger to Job and said, "The oxen were plowing and the donkeys feeding beside them, and the Sabeans fell upon them and took them and struck down the servants with the edge of the sword, and I alone have escaped to tell you." While he was yet speaking, there came another and said, "The fire of God fell from heaven and burned up the sheep and the servants and consumed them, and I alone have escaped to tell you." While he was yet speaking, there came another and said, "The Chaldeans formed three groups and made a raid on the camels and took them and struck down the servants with the edge of the sword, and I alone have escaped to tell you." While he was yet speaking, there came another and said, "Your sons and daughters were eating and drinking wine in their oldest brother's house, and behold, a great wind came across the wilderness and struck the four corners of the house, and it fell upon the young people, and they are dead, and I alone have escaped to tell you."

Then Job arose and tore his robe and shaved his head and fell on the ground and worshiped. And he said, "Naked I came from my mother's womb, and naked shall I return. The LORD gave, and the LORD has taken away; blessed be the name of the LORD."

In all this Job did not sin or charge God with wrong. "Job 1:13-22 (ESV)

Job is such a good model for how to respond in times of suffering. He did not get angry with God, he did not curse God, he instead praised God. Job had a faith that surpassed circumstances. His faith was strong and was not tossed around with the unpredictable waves of life. His faith was built on a solid foundation.

In the last part of the chapter, we will see that God is ultimately in control of our physical health. Sometimes He will allow sickness and illness in our lives for a higher purpose:

"Again there was a day when the sons of God came to present themselves before the LORD, and Satan also came among them to present himself before the LORD. And the LORD said to Satan, "From where have you come?" Satan answered the LORD and said, "From going to and fro on the earth, and from walking up and down on it." And the LORD said to Satan, "Have you considered my servant Job, that there is none like him on the earth, a blameless and upright man, who fears God and turns away from evil? He still holds fast his integrity, although you incited me against him to

destroy him without reason." Then Satan answered the LORD and said, "Skin for skin! All that a man has he will give for his life. But stretch out your hand and touch his bone and his flesh, and he will curse you to your face." And the LORD said to Satan, "Behold, he is in your hand; only spare his life."

So Satan went out from the presence of the LORD and struck Job with loathsome sores from the sole of his foot to the crown of his head. And he took a piece of broken pottery with which to scrape himself while he sat in the ashes.

Then his wife said to him, "Do you still hold fast your integrity? Curse God and die." But he said to her, "You speak as one of the foolish women would speak. Shall we receive good from God, and shall we not receive evil?" In all this Job did not sin with his lips." Job 2:1-10 (ESV)

In a very short period of time, Job encountered a magnitude of suffering that few of us will ever experience in our lifetime. Everything on this earth was taken from him. He grieved deeply, but not without hope.

The remainder of this book of the Bible details Job working through the grieving process with his friends. His friends offer him erroneous and unhelpful insights and advice. Finally, God speaks. He explains that His ways are higher than ours and we cannot fully understand His ways.

"Where were you when I laid the foundation of the earth?

Tell me, if you have understanding. Who determined its measurements—surely you know! Or who stretched the line upon it? On what were its bases sunk, or who laid its cornerstone, when the morning stars sang together and all the sons of God shouted for joy? "Or who shut in the sea with doors when it burst out from the womb, when I made clouds its garment and thick darkness its swaddling band, and prescribed limits for it and set bars and doors, and said, 'Thus far shall you come, and no farther, and here shall your proud waves be stayed'?

"Have you commanded the morning since your days began, and caused the dawn to know its place, that it might take hold of the skirts of the earth, and the wicked be shaken out of it? It is changed like clay under the seal, and its features stand out like a garment. From the wicked their light is withheld, and their uplifted arm is broken.

"Have you entered into the springs of the sea, or walked in the recesses of the deep? Have the gates of death been revealed to you, or have you seen the gates of deep darkness? Have you comprehended the expanse of the earth? Declare, if you know all this." Job 38:4–18 (ESV)

God responds to Job in a way one would not expect. An initial response might be that God is harsh and unloving toward Job. Here is how Paul Tripp continues his summary of the book of Job:

"The last four chapters of Job say, 'You're not like me. You don't know what I know. You can't do what I can do... My glory is beyond what you can understand...I'm good, I'm holy, I'm righteous, and I will do what I will. And hope is found in placing your trust in me.'"

Many times, God allows suffering so that we can see Him for the powerful, sovereign God that He is. A sovereign God whose knowledge far exceeds our own that we can trust with our lives. Famous theologian, J.I. Packer, once said:

"And still He seeks the fellowship of His people and sends them both joy and sorrow to detach their hands from the things of this world and attach those hands to Him."

Suffering in this life puts everything in the right perspective. It takes our hands off the temporary things of this world and attaches them to the only thing that can truly satisfy. God loves us and He knows what is best for us. He knows what will bring us joy. During seasons of suffering, it can feel like we have been abandoned by God. It is easy to believe that He is not the loving, gracious God that the Bible claims He is. But that might be because we are unable to see what He can see or understand what He understands.

It is so interesting how our family structure here on earth mirrors the relationship between God and us. In the Bible, God is referred to as a Father and we are His children. It was not until I had children of my own that I truly came to understand the depth and breadth of God's love for us. There are numerous times as a parent that we must either allow our children to suffer or withhold something that our children desire, to ultimately bring about good in their lives.

Our sweet toddler loves to help Mark and me around the house. He takes such pride in himself when we tell him, "Good job buddy!" One thing he loves more than anything are power tools, especially the power drill. Whenever Mark allows Drew to help him with home projects, he puts extremely strict and precise boundaries around the power tools. As the project begins, Drew quickly realizes that he cannot, for example, grab the drill by himself and turn it on. When this happens, and Mark corrects him, he falls on the ground crying. He does not understand. In his mind, Mark is a harsh, unloving father who is saying "no" to what he is sure will bring him happiness. There is no way for

Mark to explain the "why" to Drew because his brain is not able to comprehend the reasoning.

It is the same with us and God. God's ways are far higher than ours. His knowledge and understanding go beyond what our brains can comprehend. When suffering comes into our lives, we are not able to see the full picture that God can see. We are like toddlers trying to understand our Father's ways. It is impossible. The only option we have is to trust that God is a Father who loves us more than we can fathom.

When speaking on prayer, well-known apologist and teaching pastor, Tim Keller, once said:

"In short, God will either give us what we ask, or He will give us what we would have asked if we knew everything He knew."

We will not understand the "why" of every circumstance that God allows into our lives. But one thing we can do is trust that God is for us, and there is a reason for all the suffering we may encounter in this life.

Another reason for suffering in a Christian's life has to do with our hearts. Every person on this earth is born with an innate desire to go against God's commands; against what is best for them. None of us are completely good, which is why we need Jesus. The Bible teaches that this always leads to difficulties in life.

This is easily seen as we live our lives. When we give into the pride, anger, and hatred that is inherently in all our hearts, life goes bad for us. God loves us too much to allow these things to remain in our hearts and act as the driving force of our lives. God will work in us the process of sanctification, which is the process of ridding us of the sin in our hearts. 1 Thessalonians 4:3 says "For this is the will of God, your sanctification…" God's aim for His children is to use the events and circumstances in our lives to make us more like Jesus, which ultimately leads to the most joy and freedom possible in this life.

> *"Count it all joy, my brothers, when you meet trials of various kinds, for you know that the testing of your faith produces steadfastness. And let steadfastness have its full effect, that you may be perfect and complete, lacking in nothing." James 1:2-4 (ESV)*

God has a bigger aim for our lives. When life is going well, it is easy to feel like we do not need God. We can become puffed up with pride and begin to think that we did something to cause the good in our life. Pride is a sin that can destroy us from the inside out.

On the other hand, when suffering strikes, we are brought down to our knees. We are humbled. We realize how fragile we are and how dependent we are on God.

The true focus and love of our hearts are revealed, and we are sanctified and matured in our faith.

God's ultimate aim for our lives is to glorify Him and point others to Him. Sanctification is one way of doing this. When others see the way our hearts are softened and our lives take on new meaning, they can see the powerful work of God in our lives. The more our hearts are sanctified, the more joyful we become, and the more God is glorified in our lives. As pastor John Piper says, "God is most glorified in us when we are most satisfied in Him."

The final reason we suffer according to the Bible is due to the broken nature of the world. Jesus makes it clear that we will experience difficulties in this fallen world:

> *"I have told you these things, so that in me you may have peace. In this world you will have trouble. But take heart! I have overcome the world." John 16:33 (NIV)*

Nobody knew trouble and suffering better than the disciples. When they were chosen to follow Jesus, they had the understanding that Jesus, as the chosen Messiah, would be a king. That he would be the one to overthrow the ruling force of Rome. After His crucifixion and resurrection, they would soon discover that following Jesus was not going to be the life of ease that they most likely anticipated.

Following Jesus' death, the Roman and Jewish leaders began pursuing and killing those who were followers of Jesus. They were ruthless. The disciples endured horrendous suffering, including beatings, imprisonment, public stonings, crucifixion, and being boiled in oil. Paul, a Jewish convert to Christianity and leader of the early church, said in the book of 2 Corinthians:

"For we do not want you to be unaware, brothers, of the affliction we experienced in Asia. For we were so utterly burdened beyond our strength that we despaired of life itself." 2 Corinthians 1:8 (ESV)

Followers of Jesus will always suffer in this life, some far more than others. The world we live in is opposed to the message of Christianity and we should expect the world to act accordingly.

Sometimes suffering in this broken, fallen world looks like persecution. But sometimes it can look like disease, illness, accidents, broken relationships, and hatred. In a mini sermon by John Piper entitled, "Your Best Life Won't Come Now." he said:

"We are not entitled to a pain-free, trouble-free life. And getting this clear will ease the collision between expectations and reality. One of the great causes of sadness in human life is the collision of expectations and what actually happens. And the New Testament, therefore, for our joy, is relentlessly helping us to lower our expectations for this life and raise our expectations for the next. For example, in 1 Peter 4:12 it says, 'Do not be surprised at the fiery ordeal that comes upon you as though something strange were happening to you.'

In other words, get it fixed in your head that it is not strange for life to go bad for you as a Christian. And Paul in Romans 8 said, 'Even we who have the Holy Spirit groan inwardly as we wait for our adoption as children...the redemption of our bodies.' So even those, in this life, who have the Holy Spirit will experience all the rheumatism, and cancer, and accidents, and horrors that the rest of the world does. Many are the afflictions of the righteous, but the Lord delivers him out of them all.

So, the constant lowering of expectation now is accompanied with a raising of expectations later... Now we know it is going to be hard, many are the afflictions of the righteous, but oh how the New Testament raises higher and higher and higher our expectations of the life to come."

In the midst of the broken world, the apostle Paul offers us hope in the book of Romans:

"And we know that in all things God works for the good of those who love him, who have been called according to his purpose" Romans 8:28 (NIV)

God works all things, even the worst things, together for our good. Suffering in this life allows our hearts to be softened and our hands to be opened. It makes us more compassionate, more loving, and gives us a proper perspective.

We can count our suffering as joy because we know suffering allows us to see God as the compassionate, loving Father that He is.

A Father who yearns for our hearts and our hands to be free from the things of this world. Therefore, we should cling tightly to the hope and promises that only He can offer.

Chapter Ten

Let it Go My Soul and Trust in Him

Comparison was a difficult struggle to overcome during my journey. It was so difficult to see others getting the things I always wanted but never received. It was especially difficult when those people acted as though they did something to get the good they received in life. The book of Psalms is a great companion during times of struggle. King David says in Psalm 73:

> *"For I envied the arrogant when I saw the prosperity of the wicked. They have no struggles; their bodies are healthy and strong. They are free from common human burdens; they are not plagued by human ills. Therefore pride is their necklace; they clothe themselves with violence. From their callous hearts comes iniquity;*

their evil imaginations have no limits. They scoff, and speak with malice; with arrogance they threaten oppression. Their mouths lay claim to heaven, and their tongues take possession of the earth. Therefore their people turn to them and drink up waters in abundance. They say, "How would God know? Does the Most High know anything?" This is what the wicked are like— always free of care, they go on amassing wealth. Surely in vain I have kept my heart pure and have washed my hands in innocence. All day long I have been afflicted, and every morning brings new punishments." Psalm 73:3-14 (NIV)

When we are so wrapped up in our difficulties and suffering, it is easy to look around and feel like everyone else has it easy. And it is true, some people will suffer more than others in this life. But we live in a broken world, and no one gets out without feeling the effects at one point or another.

God revealed a clear message to me during one of my final therapy sessions. I was in the middle of EMDR and was feeling that I couldn't handle what the future might hold. I had barely survived the last five years; I didn't know if I had the strength to endure much more.

During the vision, I felt myself being strapped onto a roller coaster. It was pitch black and I had no idea what the roller coaster would turn into. It could be a smooth ride, or it could be filled with twists and turns that would send me into a tailspin. I tried with all my might to get out. I tugged at the straps and screamed for someone to help. Then I stopped when I heard a voice saying, "Stop fighting and be still." I quickly became calm. I looked to my left and right. I saw everyone I had ever known lined up in similar cars next to me about to get on their own roller coasters. Then a light shone down onto each of their rides. Everyone's ride was full of twists, turns and flips. No one had an easy ride; they were simply different. As the ride started, I saw everyone go off on their own tracks. The track ahead of me was still dark. I looked ahead, held on tight, and said, "Okay, let's go."

The world we live in is not what it was meant to be. It is broken. Where there was supposed to be love, joy, peace, and freedom, there is, instead, hate, anger, fear, and bondage. Suffering is a part of this world. It will affect every single person. The question is not "if," but "when." I did not need to hold onto resentments when I saw a pregnant woman get what I wanted. That woman has and will suffer in her life, it would just be in a different way. There is no room for comparison, judgment, or jealousy in this life. We all have our own rides ahead of us. They will all be different in their own way, but they will all certainly be full of twists, turns, and uncertainties at one point or another.

In the early years of our marriage, my husband would frequently quote a saying to me from his years of dirt biking, "Ride your own race." When someone is in a dirt bike race, it is important that they keep their eyes fixed on their own path. It is tempting to want to look at another rider as they go by to see what path they are taking. But the moment that racer looks over at another racer, it throws their rhythm off and they can crash.

Psalm 73 continues:

> *When my heart was grieved and my spirit embittered,*
> *I was senseless and ignorant; I was a brute beast*
> *before you. Psalm 73:21-22 (NIV)*

David realizes that bitterness and resentment toward those who seem to get what we think we deserve keeps us in bondage. It turns us into self-centered, ungrateful people. We all have our own lives to lead, and we do not need the distraction of looking over at someone else's life wishing we had what they had. We are all in this together and no one really has it any better or worse than anyone else. We need one another to navigate the difficulties of this life together with compassion, love, and understanding.

This is David's conclusion:

> *"Yet I am always with you; you hold me by my right*
> *hand. You guide me with your counsel, and afterward*

you will take me into glory. Whom have I in heaven but you? And earth has nothing I desire besides you. My flesh and my heart may fail, but God is the strength of my heart and my portion forever." Psalm 73:23-26 (NIV)

Nothing on this earth can satisfy the inner longings of our hearts. Everything, from money, to security, to people can fail us. True freedom is found when we can let go of the things of this earth, trust God with our lives, and keep our eyes fixed on what comes next. He is the treasure in this life. He is where we find our strength. He is the only source of true happiness and contentment.

"Not that I am speaking of being in need, for I have learned in whatever situation I am to to be content. I know how to be brought low, and I know how to abound. In any and every circumstance, I have learned the secret of facing plenty and hunger, abundance and need. I can do all things through him who strengthens me." Philippians 4:11-13 (ESV)

One day we will stand face-to-face with Jesus and nothing in this life will matter. This life will soon pass away, and we will experience more joy than we can even fathom.

Until then, we can be content with what God gives us in this life. We do not look to others to find what we need to be content. We keep our eye focused on our loving Father.

He will give us all we need to be able to handle whatever comes into this life, trusting it will all work for our good. The one thing we can be sure of is that God is in complete control. Our lives have significance that goes far beyond just this world. All the workings of our lives are woven into a greater story for a greater purpose.

No matter how dark things get in our lives, we can all hold on to the hope that one day Jesus will return, and he will make every wrong right. The Bible says:

> *"Then I saw a new heaven and a new earth, for the first heaven and the first earth had passed away, and the sea was no more. And I saw the holy city, new Jerusalem, coming down out of heaven from God, prepared as a bride adorned for her husband. And I heard a loud voice from the throne saying, 'Behold, the dwelling place of God is with man. He will dwell with them, and they will be his people, and God himself will be with them as their God. He will wipe away every tear from their eyes, and death shall be no more, neither shall there be mourning, nor crying, nor pain anymore, for the former things have passed away." Revelation 21:1-4 (ESV)*

* * *

Time has passed since that fateful day when my dreams of normalcy were turned upside down. The day God began to start the process of tearing down my idols, bringing me to my knees, then building my faith back stronger than it was before.

Looking back, I can see His faithfulness and steadfast love that sustained us the entire time.

Claire and Drew are the best gifts Mark and I have ever received from the Lord. They bring us more joy than we could have ever thought possible, and we are thankful every day for them.

I think back to all they have been through in their short lives. These two kids are so full of joy and love. They started out so small, but their lives have already had such a big impact on this world. I believe God will use them and their stories to impact many more in their lifetime.

I thank God that our two miracles were given to us during the season of Advent. I have been reflecting on what we celebrate during this season. The day when the light broke through the darkness and brought the desperate world hope. Through the darkness and difficulties of our journey, there was always hope. There was always light in the darkness. God never left us.

Every song we sing and verse we read during the season of Advent reminds me that God never breaks His promises. We celebrate these sweet kids' birthdays with arms lifted high to the One who can do the impossible. The One who will one day make every wrong right as we walk in the freedom we were created to have.

I never wanted the story we were given. In the end, we could have gotten two healthy pregnancies and two healthy, full-term babies. We could have received what most people get. But then I think of the people we have come to know throughout our journey and the people our children's lives have touched. I consider the people who have come to know the goodness and steadfast love of the Lord through our difficulties and struggles. I think of our hearts that were sanctified and our faith that was strengthened. Those things are far better than having two healthy, full-term babies. Those things hold eternal significance that point to something greater than ourselves.

"Set your mind on things that are above..." Colossians 3:2 (ESV)

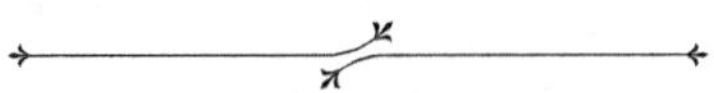

Epilogue

It is now the Fall of 2020. Claire is about to turn seven, and Drew is about to turn three. Not a day goes by that I don't marvel at how far they both have come since they entered the world.

They are the best of friends and adore one another. They truly have a special bond. They are both very protective of one another. Claire makes sure Drew is treated well when around other children, and Drew protectively shouts, "No, boy!" whenever a boy wants to play with Claire. We hope he will keep that up when she is a teenager.

Claire has done incredibly well. She met all her milestones within the normal time frame. She needed Speech Therapy for a few months when she was four years old to help her with some articulation issues. It's unknown whether her speech issues were related to her prematurity, or if she would have had them anyway. She did so well with Speech Therapy and picked it up quickly.

She is a beautiful little girl. She has blonde, flowy hair, and bright, blue eyes. She is a very smart girl. Her best subjects are math and reading comprehension. She is extremely creative and loves stories. We can see her being a writer when she grows up. She still absolutely loves kids. She is quite a bit shorter than her peers due to her prematurity, but she doesn't let that stop her. She is so outgoing and will confidently walk up to any child and introduce herself. Sometimes I envy her gregariousness. I hope she never loses that.

Drew has also done extremely well. He has met all his milestones on time (and some early). He is a rough and tumble little boy, but he also has a very sweet side. He has blonde, curly hair and dark, blue eyes. He got on the growth chart by the time he turned one and now is in the 50th percentile for height and weight (it must be all that eating he loves to do). He hasn't needed any therapies or interventions in his life.

He loves Elmo, Olaf, and anything red. He loves to be tickled and he will do just about anything to make you laugh. He is a very smart little boy. He picks up on things very quickly, and he loves to "help" Claire with her schoolwork. He can't wait to be a big boy like his daddy, who he lovingly calls, "Mawk."

Mark and I are doing very well. We still live in the house we moved into two years ago. Thankfully, our impulsiveness didn't backfire, and it turned out to be a great house in a wonderful town.

Mark still works from home as a Software Engineer. He loves being able to spend time with the kids while they are young. He is currently enjoying taking our athletic girl out on the trails to teach her to mountain bike, and teaching Drew how to fix things around the house. Both Claire and Drew look up to their daddy; he is their hero.

I am currently working at a rehab hospital as a PRN physical therapist, which means I only work occasionally. My focus is being at home and spending as much time with my sweet kids as I can. I haven't experienced any symptoms of PTSD since my last therapy session two years ago.

Our marriage is strong. We have been through so much and have found that our love grows deeper and deeper as the years pass. We look back at all we have been through and are confident that we will be able to get through anything the future may hold.

I am so grateful for my husband and my two miracle babies. Our story has made us who we are, and I wouldn't trade it for the world.

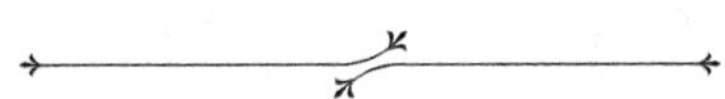

Acknowledgments

First and Foremost, I want to thank my husband, Mark, for being my best friend and greatest supporter. Thank you for giving me the encouragement to write this book.

I want to thank our OBGYN, his staff, and the NICU staff who showed such expertise, care, and compassion during our time under their care. I am confident that our babies wouldn't be here today without these people God put in our path.

Thank you to all our family and friends who supported us through our preemie journeys and the writing of this book. All of you mean so much to us and we are forever grateful for the love and guidance you gave us. Specifically, thank you to all our parents for being there any time we needed you during our five-year journey.

Thank you to my friend, Lindsey Colwill, who put so much time, effort, and care into illustrating and designing the book cover.

Last, but not least, I want to give a special thanks to Tara Tinsley. She recorded the song, "Better Early Than Never" after Claire was born, which was the inspiration for this book.